NATIONAL HEALTH CARE

NATIONAL HEALTH CARE

Law, Policy, Strategy

Donald L. Westerfield

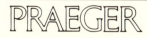

Westport, Connecticut
London

Library of Congress Cataloging-in-Publication Data

Westerfield, Donald L.
    National health care : law, policy, strategy / Donald L.
  Westerfield.
      p. cm.
    Includes bibliographical references and index.
    ISBN 0–275–94474–3 (hc : alk. paper)
    1. Insurance, Health—Law and legislation—United States.
  2. Medical care—Finance—Law and legislation—United States.
  I. Title.
  KF1183.W47   1993
  344.73′022—dc20
  [347.30422]   92–40184

British Library Cataloguing in Publication Data is available.

Library of Congress Catalog Card Number: 92–40184
ISBN: 0–275–94474–3

First published in 1993

Praeger Publishers, 88 Post Road West, Westport, CT 06881
An imprint of Greenwood Publishing Group, Inc.

Printed in the United States of America

∞™

The paper used in this book complies with the
Permanent Paper Standard issued by the National
Information Standards Organization (Z39.48–1984).

10 9 8 7 6 5 4 3 2 1

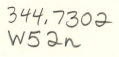
With affection, to
Mary
and to
Ronald and Douglas

There isn't a problem in the world that isn't so bad that we can't make it worse. Undoubtedly the explosion in health care costs is the most critical issue facing business and labor. The rate of increase is truly unsustainable. But if we pursue the wrong reform plan, we will do nothing to provide affordable health care to all of our people. We will instead author an economic disaster.

—Richard K. Armey (R–26–TX), before the "Oversight Hearing on National Health Care Reform," U.S. House of Representatives, 102nd Cong., 2nd Sess., 1992

Contents

Part II   Health Care Proposals in Congress

Part V   A National Health Care Plan

Figures and Tables

Figures

Tables

Preface

Our health care crisis and the spiraling costs of health care have been "front burner" issues in Congress, in the news media, and in almost every major corporate publication for the past decade. The 102nd Congress has responded with an unprecedented number of national health care plans and reform packages. Most of them, however, are more a reflection of special interest pressure to obtain favorable treatment for their own, often narrowly defined, constituencies than a carefully coordinated, nonpartisan attempt to solve the national health care crisis.

Congressional health care initiatives are clearly divided into two partisan positions on health care. The Democrats support and promote "universal" health care, to be implemented through and largely financed by the nation's employers. The Republicans support and promote "reform" measures to lighten the load on the employer while extending both the scope of health care benefits and access to them. The two views are not totally incompatible. An economically and politically feasible strategy will take the best of both concepts to formulate a national health care plan that combines comprehensive care with universal access and coverage without shifting the costs to the nation's employers.

It is largely to this end that this book was written—to present policy and strategies that cut through partisan lines to provide a basis for a national consensus on health care. The national health care plan developed in this book is nonpartisan, economically feasible, and could be implemented without causing political conflict. It was also written to be a companion to my *Mandated Health Care: Issues and Strategies*, published in 1991 by Praeger Publishers. The two books provide coverage of a wide range of health care issues and strategies with the kind of detail that is needed by policy strategists and decisionmakers at all levels of government, business and industry, and throughout the entire network of health care institutions, foundations, and scholars.

A number of members of Congress were kind enough to provide me with comments and material during the writing of this book. They include:

Representative Glen Browder (D-3-AL)

Representative Jim Cooper (D-4-TN)

Representative Ronald Dellums (D-8-CA)

Representative Thomas Downey (D-2-NY)

Representative William D. Ford (D-15-MI)

Representative Richard Gephardt (D-3-MO)

Senator John Glenn (D-OH)

Representative Henry Gonzalez (D-20-TX)

Representative Mel Hancock (R-7-MO)

Representative Joan Kelly Horn (D-2-MO)

Senator Daniel Inouye (D-HI)

Senator Edward Kennedy (D-MA)

Representative Robert Michel (R-18-IL)

Senator Sam Nunn (D-GA)

Representative Daniel Rostenkowski (D-8-IL)

Representative Jim Slattery (D-2-KS)

Representative Pete Stark (D-9-CA)

Representative Robert S. Walker (R-16-PA)

Representative Ted Weiss (D-17-NY)

I would like to thank Senator Sam Nunn (D-GA) and Senator David Pryor (D-AR) for taking the time to draft very comprehensive responses to my letters to them. I am grateful to Chairman Daniel Rostenkowski (D-8-IL) for providing me with testimony of some 85 witnesses before his "Long-Term Strategies for Health Care" hearings (102–33) in the Committee on Ways and Means. I am also grateful to Chairman William D. Ford (D-15-MI) for providing me with testimony of 11 witnesses before his "Oversight Hearing on National Health Care Reform" hearings (102–104) in the Committee on Education and Labor. Dr. Edwin Feulner, President, Heritage Foundation, was kind enough to provide me with *Heritage Foundation Backgrounders* and other material.

Additionally, the Congressional Offices of Senator Christopher Bond, Representative William Clay, Senator John Danforth, Representative Richard Gephardt, and Representative Joan Kelly Horn were especially responsive in helping me obtain bills from the U.S. House of Representatives and the U.S. Senate. Daniel P. Heslin, Corporate Director, Employee Benefit Programs, Rockwell International Corporation, provided a copy of his statement before the House Ways and Means Committee.

Two friends, who have been a constant source of encouragement and research material, are Dr. James Brasfield, Professor in the Graduate School of Webster University, and Paul Wilson, CPCU–CEBS, General Manager and Secretary-Treasurer of North American Benefit Administrators and President of NAEDA Financial Services. Jim spent hours with me discussing the political implications of health care policy and strategy. Paul has been a constant source of up-to-date health care data and counsel on health care insurance policy and strategy. Literally, I could not have completed this book without their support.

Ronald Westerfield provided research backup, designed the congressional data base for the letters to Congress and produced the final graphics. Mary Westerfield and Dr. James Brasfield proofread the manuscript. Dr. Earl Henry, Professor at Webster University, provided constant help with my transition to WordPerfect. My special thanks to them for their help in these areas.

A number of hospital administrators, underwriters, actuaries, political analysts, and scholars have provided suggestions and criticism regarding the material in this book and their views are reflected throughout the book. Staff at the Webster University Library, Saint Louis Library, and the Washington University Medical School Library have assisted me in obtaining obscure articles and material needed for the research reflected in the Bibliography.

Jim Dunton, Editor-in-Chief, at Praeger Publishers and Penny Sippel, Production Editor, at Greenwood Publishing Group were sources of both encouragement and direction for this project. I am especially grateful to them for their help and counsel.

Part I

National Health Care Issues

1

Introduction

America is facing a health care crisis. "Health care currently consumes 1 of every 8 dollars of our total production and, by the year 2000, will consume 1 of every 6 dollars."[1] As shown in Figure 1.1, our national health care expenditures are projected to be over $1.5 trillion! Our current approximate $700 billion expenditure by the health care sector has been unable to adequately care for the needs of the young poor, the unemployed, or the part-time worker. The problem is particularly acute for the predominantly part-time teenage workers, the teenage unemployed, and most single minorities.

As shown in Figure 1.2, 25.6 percent of the uninsured are children under the age of 18; 19 percent of the uninsured are teenagers and young adults aged 18 to 24 years; 25.7 percent of the uninsured are women aged 25 to 64—their most productive years; 28.7 percent of the uninsured are men also aged 25 to 64—their most productive years; and surprising to many, 0.9 percent of the uninsured are those persons who are aged 65 and over.[2]

While the figure does not give a breakdown of the categories of the uninsured, we will later find that there is a great ethnic disparity between the uninsured in almost all of the categories presented in the figure. Additionally, even though the Elderly 65 + category represents only about 1% of the total uninsured, among those who are insured there are gaps in the coverage that they experience. One important characteristic of those gaps is the requirement to "spend down" to Medicaid levels in order to have uninterrupted coverage in some cases.[3]

Figure 1.1 National Health Care Expenditures

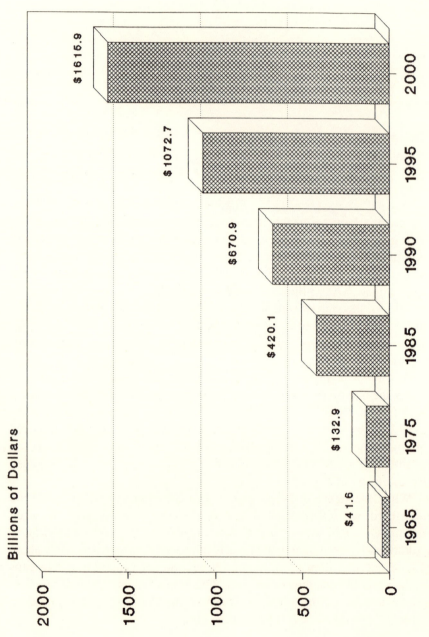

Billions of Dollars

2000		$1615.9
1995		$1072.7
1990		$670.9
1985		$420.1
1975		$132.9
1965		$41.6

Source: Health Care Financing Review, 13:1, Table 6.

Figure 1.2 Uninsured Persons as Percentage of All Uninsured Persons, 1990

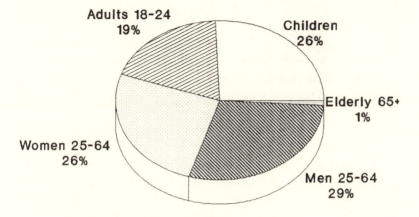

Source: "Selected Options for Expanding Health Insurance Coverage" (Washington, D.C.: Congressional Budget Office, 1991), p. xii.

Figure 1.3 Family Structure of Uninsured as Percentage of All Uninsured Persons, 1990

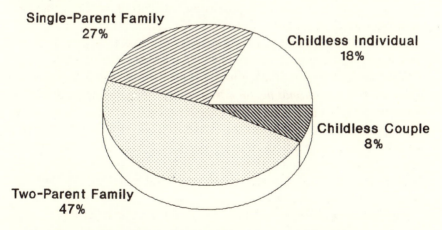

Source: "Selected Options for Expanding Health Insurance Coverage" (Washington, D.C.: Congressional Budget Office, 1991), p. xii.

Without going deeply into the demographics of the uninsured (we do that in the next chapter) it is appropriate at this point to see just how the family structure is represented in the uninsured. Figure 1.3 presents somewhat dramatic evidence of the inadequacy of the present health care system, with Childless Individuals comprising 17.9 percent of the uninsured, Single-Parent Families making up 27.2 percent of the uninsured, a surprising 47.1 percent of the uninsured being Two-Parent Families, and 7.8 percent being Childless Couples.[4]

Alarming, but expected, is the Single-Parent Family category, which comprises 27.2 percent of the uninsured. In this category we most frequently find a working female who is making just above the poverty level and does not want to become a welfare recipient. Even though her income may be above the poverty level, the prospects for sound ''well baby'' medical care are minimal, and contact with the health care delivery system may be only through the emergency room of a hospital.[5]

Probably the single most important category of the uninsured is the two-parent family, comprising about 47.1 percent of all uninsured. This family may have two working parents, but since they find themselves uninsured, their jobs are probably low-paying jobs with very few or no benefits. There could be several children in this family, all of whom will also be uninsured. Contact with the health care delivery system is usually only through the emergency room of a hospital or clinic.

This family will typically use ''home remedies'' to handle most small medical emergencies, and the efficacy and appropriateness of such remedies is directly related to the ingenuity and insights of the family member administering them. Based on typical profiles of families in the 1990 Current Population Survey, one may infer also that teenagers in such a family will typically have part-time jobs for which there are no benefits.[6]

What we see from this quick glimpse of the data regarding the uninsured is that *there is a national health care problem* for a major proportion of our population. Congress has been unable to come to grips with the scope of the problem—both how to finance and implement its solution.[7] There have been conflicting proposals in both the U.S. House of Representatives and the U.S. Senate. Some of the major health care proposals offered by those bodies of Congress are presented in Table 1.1, U.S. House of Representatives and Table 1.2, U.S. Senate.

Some of the bills cited in Tables 1.1 and 1.2 are quite lengthy and go into considerable detail in specifying the boundaries of the bills' jurisdiction. Like most projects accomplished by a committee, what started out looking like a horse turned out looking like a camel. It has four legs, a mouth, two eyes, and a tail, but it no longer serves its original purpose well, and looks a lot different from what any member of the committee had envisioned at the outset of the project. Two concepts tend not to be stated clearly in the bills—comprehensive benefits and universal access. The reason is clear. Congress knows that the American people want both

Table 1.1
Major U.S. House of Representatives Health Care Bills

Number	Short Title	Sponsor
H.R. 1	Civil Rights and Women's Equity in Employment Act of 1991	Brooks
H.R. 8	Comprehensive Health Care Act	Oakar
H.R. 16	National Health Insurance Act	Dingell
H.R. 1177	Pepper Commission Health Care Access and Reform Act of 1991	Rockefeller
H.R. 1227	HealthAmerica: Affordable Health Care for All Americans Act	Mitchell
H.R. 1270	American Family Protection Act of 1991	Stenholm
H.R. 1300	Universal Health Care Act of 1991	Russo
H.R. 1626	Employee Leave Act of 1991	LaFalce
H.R. 1669	Improvements to the HealthAmerica Act of 1991	Simon
H.R. 1777	Medicare Universal Coverage Expansion Act of 1991	Gibbons
H.R. 1872	Better Access to Affordable Health Care Act of 1991	Bentsen
H.R. 1936	Health Equity and Access Improvement Act of 1991	Chafee
H.R. 2114	Comprehensive Health Insurance Plan of 1991	Packwood
H.R. 2121	Health Insurance Reform Act of 1991	Stark
H.R. 2297	State Health Reform Opportunity Act of 1991	Markey
H.R. 2453	Small Employer Health Insurance Incentive Act of 1991	Chandler
H.R. 2530	National Health Care and Cost Containment Act	Sanders
H.R. 2535	Pepper Commission Health Care Access and Reform Act of 1991	Waxman
H.R. 3037	Health Care Liability Reform and Quality of Care Improvement Act of 1991	Archer
H.R. 3205	Health Insurance Coverage and Cost Containment Act of 1991	Rostenkowski
H.R. 3535	USHealth Program Act of 1991	Roybal

Table 1.1 (continued)

H.R. 3626	Health Insurance Reform and Cost Control Act of 1991	Rostenkowski
H.R. 5325	Action Now Health Care Reform Act of 1992	Michel
H.R. 5450	To Repeal the Americans with Disabilities Act of 1990	Edwards
H.R. 5502	Health Care Cost Containment and Reform Act of 1992	Stark

---

Source: U.S. House of Representatives

comprehensive benefits and universal access, but are unwilling to pay their costs. The compromise, therefore, is to place restrictions on both benefits and access or to shift much of the responsibility for their cost to the private sector, namely to employers.

The major impediment to reaching a national consensus on health care has been the jealous guarding of turf by the hundreds of special interests. The medical lobbies have fought any system for which fees may be standardized and for which managed care and utilization review programs oversee their activities. They favor employer-based systems, since restrictions on their services may be negotiated more easily than with Congress. Other lobbies representing those who provide medical and health care services would like to see America move closer to universal access, but want the system employer-based so that government will not be as likely to place caps on their prices and review their activities. This is the dilemma faced by Congress—how to placate the lobbies and still look like a reasonable attempt is being made to provide a solution to our health care crisis.

The U.S. Senate and U.S. House of Representatives bills, as well as other plans to be discussed later, may be classified into one of the following broad classifications of access to health care:[8]

1. National health care or single payor in each state—these are government-administered plans in which a person typically is given health care upon presentation of a national or state health care identification card.[9]
2. Mandated employer-based coverage—these plans are provided through the employers, usually with some sort of tax incentives for participation or tax disincentives for non-participation (the "play or pay" concept).[10]

Table 1.2
Major U.S. Senate Health Care Bills

Number	Short Title	Sponsor
S. 314	Comprehensive Health Care Act of 1991	Cohen
S. 454	Health Care Act	McConnell
S. 700	American Health Security Act of 1991	Durenberger
S. 1123	Health Care Liability Reform and Quality Care Improvement Act of 1991	Hatch
S. 1177	Pepper Commission Health Care Access and Reform Act of 1991	Rockefeller
S. 1211	MEDICAID Glideslope Act of 1991	Graham
S. 1227	HealthAmerica: Affordable Health Care for All Americans Act	Mitchell
S. 1229	Small Employer Health Insurance Incentive Act of 1991	McCain
S. 1446	Health USA Act of 1991	Kerry
S. 1669	Improvements to the HealthAmerica Act of 1991	Simon
S. 1872	Better Access to Affordable Health Care Act of 1991	Bentsen
S. 1936	Health Equity and Access Improvement Act of 1991	Chafee
S. 1972	State Care: State-Based Comprehensive Health Care Act of 1991	Leahy
S. 1995	Health Care Access and Affordability Act of 1991	Specter
S. 2036	Access to Health Care for All Americans Act of 1991	Kasten
S. 2114	Comprehensive Health Insurance Plan of 1991 (CHIP)	Packwood

Source: U.S. Senate

3. Expansion of Medicaid and or Medicare— typically, these plans have some tie-in with the mandated employer-based coverage. Medicaid would be the main vehicle for providing a health care "safety net" for the poor and unemployed.[11]
4. Market-based or consumer-driven—these plans typically propose tax incentives to purchase private health care plans, expansion of federal and state programs for the poor and unemployed, and removal of state mandates on health care benefits.[12]

Amid the chaos in national health care policy and in some of the proposed legislation listed in Tables 1.1 and 1.2, there are some workable strategies which must receive national consideration. The nation must consider both health care rationing and some type of multi-tier system of health care delivery.[13]

The conflict among the courts, legislators, health care providers, insurers, and other stakeholders in national health care has virtually paralyzed our national delivery system. With about 35 million persons uninsured or underinsured, the problems have become so intense that every national political candidate for Congress and for the presidency of the United States has admitted that our health care system is currently in a state of crisis, needing a national consensus which can be formulated into a national strategy for medical and health care.

Before leaving this chapter, it should be pointed out that it is remarkable that none of the bills presented in Tables 1.1 or 1.2 discuss ways in which to reform the Workers Compensation system and integrate the medical and health care portions of that system into a national health care system. Being autonomous, state-run systems, conflict caused by an injury which may be covered under Workers Compensation versus being covered under the employer's health care plan is costly and causes duplicated resources. Between 1972, when the major statewide system modifications were last made, and 1987, total costs for Workers Compensation had risen from $5.8 billion to $38 billion and the cost per employee rose from $93 to $430 during that period.[14] We go into this problem more deeply in a subsequent chapter.

The remainder of this book will present analyses of the problem, the laws and policies which relate to the problem and some sort of solution, and strategies for implementing a national health care plan.

NOTES

1. Gail Wilensky, "Cost Containment Overview," *Health Care Financing Review: 1991 Annual Supplement* (Baltimore, Md.: Health Care Financing Administration, 1991); see also, Congressional Budget Office, "Trends in Health Expenditures by Medicare and the Nation" (Washington, D.C.: CBO, 1991); Congressional Budget Office, *Rising Health Care Costs: Causes, Implications, and Strategies* (Washington, D.C.: CBO, 1991).

2. Congressional Budget Office, *Selected Options for Expanding Health Insurance Coverage* (Washington, D.C.: Congressional Budget Office, 1991), p. xii.

3. See Katharine Levit and Kathy Cowan, "Burden of Health Care Costs: Business, Households, and Government," *Health Care Financing Review* 12(2):127–137, HCFA Pub. No. 03316 (Washington, D.C.: HCFA, 1990); chapter 3 in Karen Davis and Cathy Schoen, *Health and the War on Poverty: A Ten-Year Appraisal* (Washington, D.C.: The Brookings Institution, 1978); Lester Sobel, ed., *Health Care: An American Crisis* (New York: Facts on File, Inc., 1976).

4. Congressional Budget Office, *Selected Options for Expanding Health Insurance Coverage*, 1991, *op. cit.*

5. David Eddy, "Rationing by Patient Choice," *Journal of the American Medical Association* 265 (1991):105–108; Jack Hadley, Earl Steinberg, and Judith Feder, "Comparison of Uninsured and Privately Insured Hospital Patients: Condition on Admission, Resource Use, and Outcome," *Journal of the American Medical Association* 265 (January 16, 1991):374–379.

6. Jill Foley, "Uninsured in the United States: The Nonelderly Population without Health Insurance" *Employee Benefit Research Institute Special Report SR-10* (April 1991); see also Eugene Moyer, "A Revised Look at the Number of Uninsured Americans," *Health Affairs* (Summer 1989):102–110.

7. Donald Westerfield, *Mandated Health Care: Issues and Strategies* (New York: Praeger, 1991), especially chapter 2.

8. Robert Huefner and Margaret Battin, eds., *Changing to National Health Care: Ethical and Policy Issues.* (Salt Lake City, Utah: University of Utah Press, 1992).

9. See discussions of the following bills in subsequent chapters: U.S. Senate, "Health USA Act of 1991," S. 1446, 102d Cong., 1st Sess. (Washington, D.C.: U.S. Government Printing Office, 1991); U.S. House of Representatives, "Universal Health Care Act of 1991," H.R. 1300, 102d Cong., 2nd Sess. (Washington, D.C.: U.S. Government Printing Office, 1992); U.S. House of Representatives, "Comprehensive Health Care for All Americans Act" (Claude Pepper Comprehensive Health Care Act) H.R. 8, 102d Cong., 1st Sess. (Washington, D.C.: U.S. Government Printing Office, 1991); U.S. House of Representatives, "National Health Insurance Act," H.R. 16, 102d Cong., 1st Sess. (Washington, D.C.: U.S. Government Printing Office, 1991).

10. U.S. House of Representatives, "Pepper Commission Health Care Access and Reform Act of 1991," H.R. 2535, 102d Cong., 1st Sess. (Washington, D.C.: U.S. Government Printing Office, 1991); U.S. House of Representatives, "USHealth Program Act of 1991," H.R. 3535, 102d Cong., 2nd Sess. (Washington, D.C.: U.S. Government Printing Office, 1992); U.S. Senate, "Pepper Commission Health Care Access and Reform Act of 1991," S. 1177, 102d Cong., 1st Sess. (Washington, D.C.: U.S. Government

Printing Office, 1991); U.S. Senate, "HealthAmerica: Affordable Health Care for All Americans Act," S. 1227, 102d Cong., 1st Sess. (Washington, D.C.: U.S. Government Printing Office, 1991); U.S. Senate, "Comprehensive Health Insurance Plan of 1991 (CHIP of 1991)," S. 2114, 102d Cong., 1st Sess. (Washington, D.C.: U.S. Government Printing Office, 1991).

11. The bills are combinations of reform and state plan bills cited throughout chapters 5 through 7 of this book; for example, U.S. Senate, "State Care: State-Based Comprehensive Health Care Act of 1991," S. 1972, 102d Cong., 1st Sess. (Washington, D.C.: U.S. Government Printing Office, 1991).

12. Most of these proposals are "reform" proposals contained in U.S. House of Representatives, "Health Insurance Reform and Cost Control Act of 1991," H.R. 3626, 102d Cong., 2nd Sess. (Washington, D.C.: U.S. Government Printing Office, 1992); U.S. Senate, "Comprehensive Health Care Act of 1991," S. 314, 102d Cong., 1st Sess. (Washington, D.C.: U.S. Government Printing Office, 1991); U.S. Senate, "American Health Security Act of 1991," S. 700, 102d Cong., 1st Sess. (Washington, D.C.: U.S. Government Printing Office, 1991); U.S. Senate, "Health Care Liability Reform and Quality Care Improvement Act of 1991," S. 1123, 102d Cong., 1st Sess. (Washington, D.C.: U.S. Government Printing Office, 1991); U.S. Senate, "Better Access to Affordable Health Care Act of 1991," S. 1872, 102d Cong., 1st Sess. (Washington, D.C.: U.S. Government Printing Office, 1991); U.S. Senate, "Health Equity and Access Improvement Act of 1991," S. 1936, 102d Cong., 1st Sess. (Washington, D.C.: U.S. Government Printing Office, 1991).

13. Stephen Jencks and George Schieber, "Containing U.S. Health Care Costs: What Bullet to Bite?" *Health Care Financing Review: 1991 Annual Supplement* (Baltimore, Md.: Health Care Financing Administration, 1992); "The Crisis in Health Insurance," *Consumer Reports* (Aug. 1990):533–549; L. R. Churchill, *Rationing Health Care In America: Perceptions And Principles Of Justice* (Notre Dame, In.: University of Notre Dame Press, 1987).

14. Casey Young and Phillip Polakoff, "Beyond Workers' Compensation: A New Vision" *Benefits Quarterly* (3rd Quarter 1992):56–65; National Commission on State Workmen's Compensation Laws, *The Report of the National Commission on State Workmen's Compensation Laws* (Washington, D.C.: U.S. Government Printing Office, 1972); Jerry Miccolis, "Workers' Compensation—The State of the System" *Emphasis* (1991/1992):15–17; U.S. Chamber of Commerce, *1990 Analysis of Workers' Compensation Laws* (Washington, D.C.: U.S. Chamber of Commerce, 1991).

2

The Uninsured and Underinsured

With approximately 34.4 million persons under the age of 65 uninsured and millions more underinsured, "16 percent of the population under 65 are uninsured. For minority populations, the statistics are worse—for example, 21.7 percent of blacks are uninsured, and 34.9 percent of Mexican Americans are uninsured."[1] It is remarkable that there has been no real progress in access to health care in the most current decade.[2] It is not common knowledge that millions of workers are not covered by any kind of health care plan. It is also not common knowledge that even workers with health care plans often cannot afford to get health care, due to the high "up front" deductible.[3]

A person who is making between $20,000 and $30,000 with a non-working spouse and any children will have a hard time just trying to scrape up even $50 to $75 for some office visits, plus at least that much for the prescribed medicine. Additionally, many of those with marginal incomes find that they have to face staggering costs associated with complications such as underweight and/or critically ill babies, indigent dependents, and family members with chronic illnesses or conditions, just to name a few. Such costs, even for families with moderate incomes can be devastating to the family financial structure.[4]

A good example of the plight even people with insurance face is tragically illustrated in the case of Ann Krame of Saint Louis and her son, Stephen, who had a 14-hour operation to rebuild his pulmonary artery system. "Stephen's six-month hospital stay cost more than

$800,000, and that doesn't include doctors' fees, said Ann Krame. A recent ventilator bill was nearly $4,000; a monitor to record her son's oxygen level costs $700 a month. Ann Krame calculates Stephen's medical bills total well over $1.5 million. They have exceeded the $1 million limit on her husband's insurance policy. Stephen has been denied Medicaid coverage."[5]

The example just cited, tragic as it is, is more typical than one might imagine. The American Hospital Association estimates that there are between 17,000 and 30,000 "technologically dependent" children in this country and that about $2.6 billion is spent every year on neonatal intensive care. It is not uncommon for costs of such babies to amount to over $1 million, with the average being about $159,000 per infant.[6]

Even with insurance coverage, workers and their families are finding it increasingly difficult to cope with significant increases in premiums that seem to have no end. Larry Beddingfield was reported to be going into a "health-insurance hell" when his monthly health care premiums, to cover himself, his wife, and five children, jumped from $258 to $917.19, or $11,000 a year. His firm, Chiz Brothers, Inc., of Elizabeth, Pennsylvania, has experienced health insurance premium increases of 50 percent in the last year, to a staggering $5,220 per employee per year.[7] These types of increases are not an uncommon experience for both employees of small firms and for the small firms themselves.

If the squeeze is on the small firms and their employees, it is easy to imagine what a precarious situation it must be for the uninsured and especially the unemployed. Their health care options are meager at best.

DEMOGRAPHIC CHARACTERISTICS OF THE UNINSURED

Much of the statistical data for the uninsured and underinsured refer to the poverty threshold for given categories of individuals and families. Table 2.1 presents the weighted average poverty threshold based on money income for families and related individuals in 1989. The table indicates that the poverty threshold for a family of four in 1989 was $12,675. Compare this with the two-person under 65 years of age household figure of $8,343.[8] These are very low levels indeed. It seems that these thresholds should more correctly be called the subsistence thresholds, since it is doubtful that such income levels could support little more than a bare subsistence.

The poverty thresholds have been increasing at an annual compound

Table 2.1
Poverty Thresholds 1989

Single Childless	**$6,311**
Under 65 Years	**6,451**
65 Years and Over	**5,947**
2 Persons	**8,076**
Householder Under 65	**8,343**
Householder 65 and Over	**7,501**
3 Persons	**9,885**
4 Persons	**12,675**
5 Persons	**14,990**
6 Persons	**16,921**

Source: Bureau of the Census, "Statistical Abstract of the United States, 1991," p. 430.

rate of about 6.39 percent since 1970. What is more striking is the contrast of persons and families below the poverty level among the races. Figure 2.1 indicates that the percentage of families below the 1989 poverty level for blacks is about 3.6 times that for whites. The figure also indicates that black persons are slightly worse off than black families and the ratio of the percentage of black persons to white persons below the 1989 poverty level is 3 to 1. The percentages of all families and persons for "All Races" is slightly higher that the percentages for whites, but are disproportionately lower than the percentages for the blacks.

Contrary to what many may think about those below the poverty level, those families and individuals may not be eligible for Medicaid or Medicare. Medicaid is tied in with a state's welfare system, and that makes the eligibility for and receipt of Medicaid coverage vary by state. For

Figure 2.1 Percentages of Families and Persons Below the 1989 Poverty Level

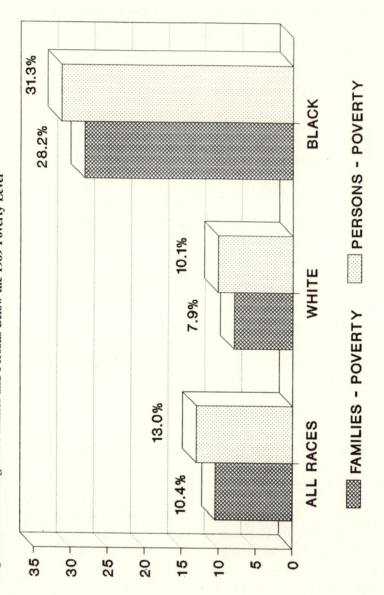

FAMILIES - POVERTY   PERSONS - POVERTY

Source: U.S. Bureau of the Census, "Statistical Abstract of the United States, 1991" (Washington, D.C.: U.S. Department of Commerce, 1991), p. 38.

example, a two-parent family with several children may be at or below the poverty level because the parents may receive minimum wages from full-time employment with an employer who may not provide health care benefits. This family may not qualify for Medicaid in a given state. Single persons who do not have dependents may not qualify for Medicaid. Additionally, students who are independent of their parents or who may be partially dependent on their parents may not qualify for Medicaid.

Table 2.2 presents some selected characteristics of uninsured persons in 1990.[9] Perhaps some of the most remarkable statistics on the uninsured from Table 2.2 are the percentages in the "Family Work Status" category: 80.2 percent of the uninsured were employed in 1990; 6.1 percent of the uninsured are unemployed; 13.7 percent of the uninsured are not even in the labor force. Informal questioning of persons interested in national health care will usually reveal that most persons believe that the uninsured are primarily the unemployed. We can see from Table 2.2 that it is just the reverse—it is the employed who make up the major proportion of the uninsured.

Women and men aged 25 to 64 years make up about a quarter of the uninsured each, with men a little worse off than women by 3 percentage points. In the previous discussion of those at or below the poverty level, a reference was made regarding the two-parent family. Notice that 47.1 percent of the uninsured are two-parent families and over a quarter of all uninsured are single-parent families (27.2 percent).

UNEMPLOYED AND UNINSURED

The data presented in Table 2.2 present a dimension of the uninsured that may be in conflict with common thinking about the uninsured. The common misconception is that the uninsured are unemployed. Both Table 2.2 and Figure 2.2 should shed new light on that matter. We see from both that the larger proportion of the uninsured are indeed employed. Figure 2.2, however, adds more detail to dispel that misconception. Notice from the figure that 54.4 percent of the uninsured have full-time jobs with no unemployment, while 8.1 percent of the uninsured have part-time jobs with no unemployment.[10] This means that about 62.5 percent of the non-elderly uninsured experienced no unemployment in 1990. The picture for the full-time and part-time job holders who experience some unemployment is quite different. They make up about 23.1 percent of the nonelderly uninsured, with 14.1 percent and 9.0 percent respectively.

Table 2.2
Characteristics of Uninsured Persons, 1990

Characteristic	Percent of All Uninsured
All Uninsured	100.0
Family Work Status:	
Employed	80.2
Unemployed	6.1
Not in Labor Force	13.7
Family Income as a Percent of Poverty Level (1989):	
Below 200	60.6
200 or Higher	39.4
Age and Sex:	
Children	25.6
Young Adults, 18 to 24	19.0
Women, 25 to 64	25.7
Men, 25 to 64	28.7
Elderly, 65 and Over	0.9
Race:	
White	77.5
Black	17.5
Other	5.0
Family Structure:	
Unrelated Individual	17.9
Single-Parent Family	27.2
Two-Parent Family	47.1
Childless Couple	7.8

Source: Selected Options for Expanding Health Insurance Coverage'' (Washington, D.C.: Congressional Budget Office, 1991), p. xii.

Figure 2.2 Nonelderly Percent of Uninsured by Employment, 1990

Percent of Uninsured by Employment Type

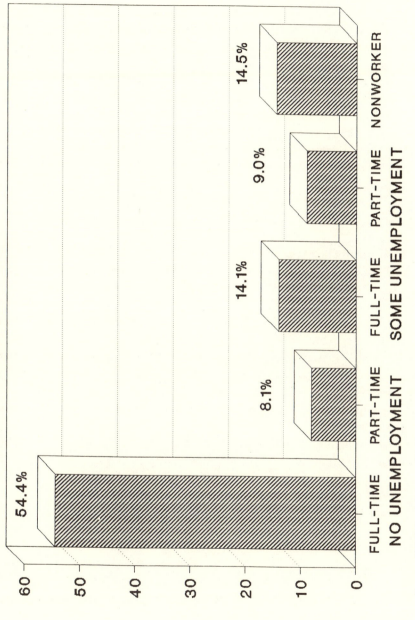

Source: ERBI Special report, SR-10, April, 1991, Table 2.

The last three categories may not be so obvious to the casual observer of the uninsured. The 14.5 percent nonelderly nonworkers consist primarily of those dependents of workers who may not have family coverage or be dependents of workers who do not have health care benefits on the job. Additionally, they do not qualify for Medicare or Medicaid because they make too much money to receive welfare and Medicaid, their family structure is such that they do not qualify for Medicaid, they may be students, or any number of other reasons.

The full-time uninsured with some unemployment could be:

Non-union workers in different trades, especially construction and the building trades

Workers working on a "contract basis" for any number of businesses

Workers in several of the service industries

Self-employed persons

Workers in industries for which there are traditionally periods of layoffs

Workers in small firms of all types (typically firms with less than 50 employees)

The list could be expanded many times, but it is sufficient to indicate the nature of the workers who might be classified as full-time, but be subject to some unemployment during the year.

Perhaps it is appropriate in discussing the unemployed and uninsured to indicate the levels of education of the nonelderly uninsured. Figure 2.3 presents a breakdown of the 1990 nonelderly uninsured by level of education.[11] It is not obvious why certain of the categories in the figure make up the given proportions of the uninsured. The jump from 16.9 percent for those with no high school and 17.4 percent for those with some high school to the 38.7 percent for high school graduates needs some explanation.

High school graduates constitute the major single proportion of the uninsured by education level in 1990. If a person graduates from high school and has to go to work immediately, it is highly likely that the first job will be an entry level or minimum wage job in a firm that does not provide health care benefits to its employees. Very often an employer will hire high school graduates for 37.5 hours per week instead of 40 hours per week so that these employees are not legally classified as full-time employees in most states. In so doing, the employer may escape the requirement to pay the part-time workers any benefits at all. This practice is very common in fast food establishments and in department stores.

Some high school graduates who never go to college get married and

Figure 2.3 Nonelderly Percent of Uninsured by Education, 1990

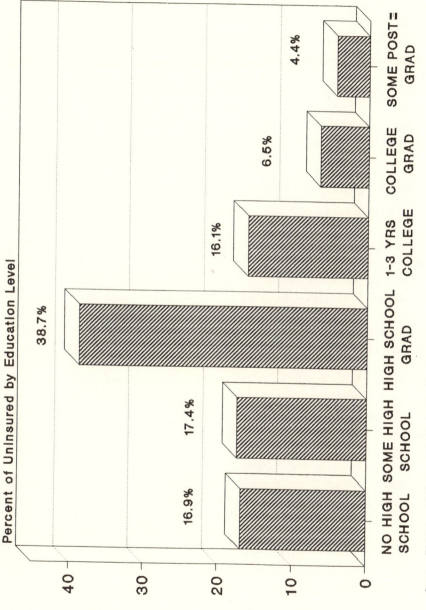

Percent of Uninsured by Education Level

16.9%   17.4%   38.7%   16.1%   6.5%   4.4%

NO HIGH   SOME HIGH   HIGH SCHOOL   1-3 YRS   COLLEGE   SOME POST≡
SCHOOL   SCHOOL   GRAD   COLLEGE   GRAD   GRAD

Source: ERBI Special Report, SR-10, April, 1991, Table 3.

become ineligible for coverage under a parent's health insurance policy. Of course, some high school graduates remain unemployed or are casual workers in some occupation. Both of these categories would generally preclude any health care coverage under a family policy or under an employer's health care plan.

The remaining three categories in Figure 2.3 involve more unemployment, part-time employment, or employment with a firm that does not provide health care benefits. For these categories of students, there is also the likelihood that age becomes a more important factor than for the other categories; that is, at age 23, most family coverage ceases even though the student is a full-time student. Between age 18 and age 23, the full-time student may be covered by the family health care plan.

MEDICAID AS A STOPGAP

In its original form, Medicaid (Title XIX of the *Social Security Amendments of 1965*) was enacted as a companion to Medicare so that the states, in combination with the federal government, could provide access to health care to certain low-income persons and groups enrolled in public assistance programs. As the Advisory Commission on Intergovernmental Relations Report of 1992 points out, using Medicaid as a "stopgap" measure to provide access to health care for a large proportion of the uninsured cannot be the best alternative to a comprehensive reform of the overall health care system in America.

Although Medicaid is a means-tested entitlement program, it has never provided coverage for all of the poor. The Census Bureau reports that 45.2 percent of the poverty population was covered by Medicaid in 1990. Moreover, many Medicaid recipients are not poor. The comparison between the number of Medicaid enrollees and the poverty population is to show relative scale only. Some Medicaid enrollees have incomes above the poverty level, especially as a result of the medically needy option and recent expansions of Medicaid to pregnant women and children up to 133 percent of poverty and higher. The Medicaid population can be classified into seven major categories:

- The elderly (age 65 and over);
- The blind;
- The disabled, defined as permanently and totally disabled, including the mentally retarded, mentally ill, and developmentally disabled;

- Dependent children under age 21, primarily those in families receiving AFDC, SSI, or defined as medically needy;
- Adults in families with dependent children;
- Pregnant women and children under age 6 in families with incomes less than 133 percent of the poverty level; and
- Other Title XIX beneficiaries, mainly children who meet income and asset requirements for cash assistance programs but do not meet the definition of dependent child (e.g., children under 21 in two-parent families).[12]

As indicated from the foregoing, any attempt to expand the Medicaid network to provide greater access will have to be worked out in at least a three-dimensional plan:

1. States will have to decide which part, or all, of the uninsured will be covered by the Medicaid safety net.
2. States will have to make qualifications for Medicaid standard across all states.
3. States will have to work out what share of the burden of the uninsured will be assumed by the state budgets versus the federal budget for the uninsured.

The alternative to the three dimensions of the problem mentioned above is that the federal government will mandate an extension of Medicaid benefits to all persons not employed and not eligible for Medicare. The federal law would supersede all state laws due to the federal "supremacy clause." This is the "single payer" concept that will be discussed in length, including an analysis of the bills advocating such a system, in a subsequent chapter.

THE UNDERINSURED

The underinsured are those who have insurance coverage, but whose insurance coverage is not adequate for their own or their dependents' health care liabilities. They would include those persons who:

1. Have basic insurance coverage, but have no major medical insurance.
2. Have basic insurance coverage, but the upper limits on in-patient care, home care, mental and drug rehabilitation, etc. have been exceeded.

3. Have indemnity policies and the per diem allowances are inadequate for the type of care needed.
4. Have coverage except for a preexisting condition. Either the plan will not cover the preexisting condition at all or the subscriber will have to wait up to 12 months before it is covered. In some plans, "pregnancy is considered a preexisting condition if full-term takes place during the first 270 days of coverage."
5. Have long-term, chronic and/or catastrophic conditions not covered by a basic plan.
6. Are on non-military leave of absence, on anticipated disability leave, or care of newborn child leave and may receive no vision or dental care or may receive only basic coverage.
7. Are laid off with less than threshold net credited service, may have no dental or vision care, and may receive only 6 months company paid benefits.
8. Go to physicians and/or clinics outside a given PPO or HMO network and may have lifetime maximums reduced to as low as $50,000.[13]

There are also many services which are not covered at all in a basic health care plan. While these services are not deemed "medically necessary," they nevertheless are necessary for a person's health and welfare. Policies which do not cover them cause a person to have to pay for them "out of pocket." Examples of some of these services are:

1. Custodial, domiciliary or sanitorium care, care in a home for the aged, care in a nursing home or convalescent home, or a skilled nursing home if the person does not qualify for Medicare.
2. Eye surgery such as keratotomy.
3. Hospitalization primarily for physical therapy or speech therapy.
4. Services rendered as a result of an injury, illness, or disease arising out of the participation in or attempt to commit a felony or assault.
5. Any charges over the reasonable and customary fees charged by specialists for a given injury or illness.

6. Most diagnostic tests unless directly related to an accident or severe inpatient episode.
7. Most organ transplants.

The non-coverage or partial coverage of these services may be potentially devastating to the finances of persons needing the services. The conditions or illnesses run their course without regard to the person's ability to pay. Equally serious consequences arise when certain diseases are not insurable in a given health care plan. Those diseases or conditions are chronic and usually result in thousands of dollars of claims over the lifetime of the person having them.

There is a tendency for health care plans of larger firms, especially those not self-insured, to cover one or more of the diseases or conditions listed below. In view of the costs involved, most small firms typically exclude the following from their health care plans:

Diabetes

Cancer and cancer-related conditions

Chronic or severe heart problems

Hypertension

Leukemia and other diseases of the blood

Rheumatoid arthritis and other chronic and severe arthritis conditions

AIDS and AIDS-related complex

Chronic back problems

Guillain-Barré

Crohn's disease

Kidney problems

Lung diseases

Chronic alcoholism and drug addiction

Diseases and conditions associated with a risky lifestyle or profession

The list could go on and on, but there are enough items listed to indicate that basic health care policies do not cover many of the diseases and conditions that result in a high dollar claims experience. While most of these conditions are excluded, riders, for individuals willing to pay for the added premium, are almost prohibitively expensive—often costing more than the base policy. The exclusions cause those with these diseases or conditions to be underinsured and among those for which a national policy must be designed.

In the following chapter we follow up the uninsured and underinsured with an analysis of the concept of underwriting "impaired risks." Who should pay for these risks? Are they primarily society's risks or individual risks? Should businesses share the burden of covering them? Answering these questions involves facing the dilemma that the public generally believes that there is a social obligation to cover impaired risks, but no acceptable plan has been designed yet to allocate their costs equitably among business, government, and individuals.

NOTES

1. Testimony of William Roper, Director, Centers for Disease Control, before the U.S. House of Representatives, *Long-Term Strategies for Health Care*, Hearings Before the Committee on Ways and Means, House of Representatives, Serial 102–33, 102d Cong., 1st Sess., April 16–17, 23–25, 1991 (Washington, D.C.: U.S. Government Printing Office, 1992), p. 18.

2. Testimony of Daniel Heslin on behalf of the ERISA Industry Committee before the U.S. House of Representatives, *Oversight Hearing on National Health Care Reform*, Serial No. 102–104, 7 May 1992 (Washington, D.C.: U.S. Government Printing Office, 1992), pp. 60–70.

3. John Holahan and Sheila Zedlewski, "Insuring Low-Income Americans Through Medicaid Expansion," Urban Institute Working Paper No. 3836–02 (December 1989); Lisa S. Howard, "Health Providers Blamed For Ranks Of Uninsureds," *National Underwriter* (Oct. 10 1988):5–6; Gail Jensen, Michael Morrisey, and John Marcus, "Cost Sharing And The Changing Pattern Of Employer-Sponsored Health Benefits," *The Milbank Quarterly* 65(4)(1987):521–550.

4. Testimony of Gilbert Omenn before the U.S. House of Representatives, *Long-Term Strategies For Health Care, op. cit.*, pp. 56–86.

5. Peter Hernon, "Critically Ill Infants Pose Sad Dilemma: Some Question Life at any Cost," *Saint Louis Post Dispatch*, 14 June 1992, pp. 1, 6.

6. Ibid.

7. Kevin Anderson, "Small Firms are Getting Squeezed Out," *USA Today*, 13 June 1991, pp.1B–2B.

8. U.S. Department of Commerce, *Statistical Abstract of the United States 1991* (Washington, D.C.: Bureau of the Census, 1991), p. 430.

9. Congressional Budget Office, *Selected Options for Expanding Health Insurance Coverage* (Washington, D.C.: U.S. Government Printing Office, 1991), p. xii.

10. Jill Foley, "Uninsured in the United States: The Nonelderly Population Without Health Insurance" Employee Benefit Research Institute (ERBI), Special Report SR-10, (April, 1991), p. 38.

11. Jill Foley, *op. cit.*, Table 3.

12. Advisory Commission on Intergovernmental Relations, *MEDICAID Intergovern-mental Trends and Options* No. A-119 (Washington, D.C.: USACIR, 1992), p. 33.

13. Blue Cross Blue Shield of Missouri, *Your Health Care Benefits with Alliance Select*, Blue Cross Blue Shield of Missouri Program Booklet, Saint Louis, Missouri, 1991, p. 8.

3

Underwriting, "Impaired Risks," and Pooling

The term "impaired risk" means a risk that is a nonstandard risk or one which would normally not be insurable except under special conditions, usually spelled out in a rider, and with an added premium to cover the added risk.[1] This term implies separating out some risks and accepting others based on claims experience or state of health of a given group or individuals. The insurance business is not entirely settled on what the concept means, but there is fairly general agreement that the thrust of the concept is to view a risk as being impaired if it is not a standard risk or is one that is usually not accepted as standard in a basic health care policy.[2]

Many of the conditions and diseases mentioned in the previous chapter would be considered as impaired risks, that is, conditions and diseases such as diabetes, cancer and cancer related conditions, chronic or severe heart problems, hypertension, leukemia and other diseases of the blood, rheumatoid arthritis and other chronic and severe arthritis conditions, AIDS and AIDS-related complex, chronic back problems, Guillain-Barré, Crohn's disease, kidney problems, chronic lung conditions and diseases, and chronic alcoholism and drug addiction.[3]

During the first 31 days of employment, some or all of these conditions and diseases may be accepted by the group plan, but thereafter they would most likely be either accepted with special conditions and a special rate or not be accepted at all by the insurer.

PREEXISTING CONDITIONS AS IMPAIRED RISKS

The "preexisting conditions" provision in a health care plan means a policy provision which excludes or limits coverage for charges or expenses incurred during a specified period (most often 3, 6, or 12 months) following the insured's effective date of coverage.[4] The term "preexisting condition" refers to a condition which, during a specified period immediately preceding the effective date of coverage, had manifested itself in such a manner as would cause an ordinarily prudent person to seek medical advice, diagnosis, or care or treatment. This would include a condition for which an insured was *recommended* to receive or *actually* received medical advice, diagnosis, or care or treatment. It also covers a pregnancy existing on the effective date of coverage under a company health care plan.

There is no uniformity regarding the treatment of preexisting conditions by a given company's health care plan. The trend now is to accept all persons enrolling in a group plan if that enrollment takes place within the first 31 days of employment. If the preexisting condition is not automatically covered in the first 31 days, it may become covered if one or more of the following criteria are met:

1. The insured has received no treatment for the preexisting condition for a period of three months after the enrollment date.
2. The insured has had perfect attendance on the job for a period of six months after the enrollment date.
3. The insured has been covered by the plan for twelve successive months in the given company.

One of the major exceptions to the above is the infectious disease AIDS. It has puzzled many underwriters and plan administrators that The Americans With Disabilities Act of 1991 has classified AIDS as a disability and not as an infectious disease, as in the case of other infectious diseases such as syphilis or ghonerrea.[5] What this effectively accomplishes is that AIDS cannot be a disqualifying underwriting consideration in a company's group health care plan. Even though it may be a preexisting condition, it cannot be treated as such under the provisions of The Americans with Disabilities Act. The Act states:

(A) PROHIBITED EXAMINATIONS AND INQUIRIES.—A covered entity shall not require a medical examination and shall not make inquiries of an employee as to whether such employee is an individual with a disability or as to the nature or severity of the disability, unless such examination or inquiry is shown to be job-related and consistent with business necessity.[6]

When we analyze some of the U.S. Senate and U.S. House of Representatives proposals for health care reform, we will find, among other things, that there is no set pattern for handling preexisting conditions. An interesting approach to preexisting conditions is set out in H.R. 3535, short title "USHealth Program Act of 1991," introduced by Representative Edward R. Roybal (D-25-CA). Secs. 2154 (b)(1–2) state, in part:

(b) Treatment of Pre-Existing Condition Exclusions for All Services.—

(1) In General.—Subject to the provisions of this subsection, a qualified health plan (other than the USHealth Program) may exclude coverage with respect to services related to treatment of a preexisting condition, but the period of such exclusion may not exceed 6 months.
(2) Nonapplication to Newborns and Sunset of Pre-Existing condition exclusions for Required Health Services.—The exclusion of coverage permitted under paragraph (1) shall not apply to—
    (A) services furnished to newborns, or
    (B) required health services furnished on or after July 1 of the 6th year beginning after the date of the enactment of this title.

Notice that the language of Sec. 2154 (b)(2)(B) would have preexisting conditions clauses expire after the sixth year after the enactment of this bill. The Rostenkowski bill, H.R. 3205, contains a similar provision, except that the "sunset" period is "July 1 of the 4th year beginning after the date of the enactment of this title."[8] Most of the other major proposals in the U.S. Senate and in the U.S House of Representatives permit exclusions for preexisting conditions in the health care plans.

For most insurance companies, the preexisting condition clause may exclude preexisting conditions for the life of the insured, *if the insured is covered under an individual policy*. In all such cases, if the insured does not buy a special policy to cover the excluded condition, this person will be included in the millions of persons who are underinsured, that is, the insurance policy is inadequate to cover all the person's health care liability.

UNDERWRITING HIGH-COST/HIGH-RISK GROUPS

The impaired risk problem is especially acute in the small group health insurance market, in which a growing number of small business owners are faced with enormous rate increases when one or more of the employees develops a major illness.[9] It is not uncommon for an insurer to take a second look at its coverage of a small group when one or more cases of AIDS appears in the most recent year's experience, especially if high claims result from advanced stages of the virus.[10]

Employers having employees with low claims experience are given more favorable rates than those employers with higher claims experience. It seems reasonable to argue that a firm with low claims should not have to pay the same rate as a firm with a high claims experience. In such a case, the firm with the more favorable experience would, in effect, be subsidizing the rates of the firm with the less favorable claims experience (or sicker employees). This is the core of the problems associated with many of the national health care plans—many of the proposed national health care plans want high-cost/high-risk groups or individuals to pay the same rate as the low cost/low risk groups or individuals through "community rates." We will discuss this type of rating proposal in depth in subsequent sections.

When the government requires insurers to take all applicants and narrow the range of rates to be charged there would be a tendency for some insurers to be the object of "adverse selection," that is, they might be stuck with a disproportionately high percentage of high-risk and high-cost groups. This could happen due to the industry, geography, line of business, etc. in which the insurer has typically been writing its business. Unless there is some mechanism for distributing high-risk/high-cost groups or individuals among several insurers, the shrewder insurers will design their business in such a manner that the low-cost, young and healthy individuals or groups are covered and the high-cost, older groups or individuals are screened out. This type strategy has often been referred to as "cream skimming" or "cherry picking."

When legislators try to implement plans in which high-cost and low-cost groups or individuals pay the same rate, at least the following two results obtain:

1. The low-cost groups or individuals will be subsidizing the high-cost groups or individuals.
2. More small employers' rates will go up than will go down,

and some currently insured groups will be caused to drop coverage.

This move to common or "community" rates does not address the cause of the problem in the first place, that of ever-increasing medical costs. In a competitive market, insurers set rates for a given group based on what the coverage is expected to cost during the next year. Any significant increase in the rates of one group to subsidize the rates of another group will have detrimental effects on the insurers' business when this "community" scheme is found out.

COMMUNITY RATING

The "Waxman Bill," H.R. 2535, with short title "Pepper Commission Health Care Access and Reform Act of 1991" contains the following language in Sec. 2231(2)(B):

Each actuarial rate shall be established in a manner so that if all eligible individuals in the class were enrolled under this title for the benefit package in the community, the aggregate of the rates would be equal to the total expenditures (including administrative expenses) with respect to that class, benefit package, and community under this title in that following year. Each such actuarial rate shall be uniform within each beneficiary class, benefit package, and community, and shall not vary among such individuals by age, sex, health, or other risk characteristics.[11]

As one might expect, this is the exact language that one will find in the Senate version of the same bill, "Rockefeller Bill," S. 1177, "Pepper Commission Health Care Access and Reform Act of 1991" with same section and subsection citations.[12] Although the language of the "Roybal Bill," H.R. 3535, "USHealth Program Act of 1991" is different from that of the Waxman and Rockefeller bills, the concept of a common rate is the foundation of the premiums. The bill states, in Section 2712(b) and (e):

(b) Use of Community-Rating.—The reference premium rate charged for an employer health plan with similar benefits in a community for a type of family enrollment (described in subsection (e)) shall be the same for all employers.

(e) Types of Family Enrollment.—Each employer health plan shall permit enrollment of (and shall compute premiums separately for) individuals based on each of the following beneficiary classes:

(A) 1 adult.

(B) A married couple without children.

(C) 1 adult and 1 child.

(D) A married couple with 1 or more children, or 1 adult with 2 or more children.[13]

Notice that in the Roybal Bill, the communities are defined in (A) through (D) above, and that the rates are the same without regard to sex, age, health status, or other underwriting characteristics. This again points out the fact that the low-cost segments of each of the communities listed above will be subsidizing the high-cost segments of the respective communities. For example, in the "1 adult" category, a healthy young worker will pay the same premium as an older sick worker, even though the costs could be different by a factor of five to ten or more per year.

If there are options that allow an employee to choose between a federal plan with community rates and an employer plan that contains rates based on underwriting characteristics, adverse selection will fill the federal plan with sicker, high-cost employees, while the employer plan will likely wind up with the healthier and younger employees at a lower cost.

For the smaller groups with under 25 employees, administrative costs amount to anywhere from 25 percent to 40 percent of the costs of health care. Costs of claims are the predominant cost. It is easy to see that high medical costs of even a few sick employees will tend to make the small group's costs per employee much higher than would be the case if they could be spread over a larger number of employees. These higher costs per employee cause that group's risk factor to increase in the eyes of an insurer.

Polzer and Jones of The George Washington University National Health Policy Forum get to the core of the community rating system's pooling of high-cost individuals with low-cost individuals in observing:

Because health care costs are dramatically higher for the sickest fraction of the population, insurance purchasers whose claim costs are expected to be low have a great incentive to avoid being pooled with customers whose claim costs are expected to be high. Each year, a relatively unpredictable 5 percent of the population incurs about half of all medical expenses; 20 percent of the population incurs about 80 percent of total medical costs, says George Berry, an actuary for Milliman & Robertson, Inc.

Put another way, the 5 percent of the U.S. population using the most health care generated expenses at least 26 times greater per capita than people at the midpoint of the distribution ($7,100 at the 95th percentile compared to $270 each at the 50th percentile in 1987), the Agency for Health Care Policy and Research reported in 1991. The ratio between the 95th percentile and the 25th percentile was far greater: 142 to 1 ($7,100 compared to $50).[14]

It is this disparity which causes debate regarding the legislative reforms and how any national health care plan will be implemented. Politicians have publicly stated that there is a growing unwillingness of middle and upper incomed persons to further subsidize the "underclass." In the light of the above contrasts, it is likely that there will be maximum resistance to implementing any national health care system which would have the appearance of transferring more burden from the sick to the healthy and from the poor to the wealthy.

SPREADING RISKS THROUGH REINSURANCE

Reinsurance, a concept discussed among underwriters and actuaries, is little known to the public and can have a significant impact on access to health insurance from small employers or small groups. Often, the projected or expected risk faced by the self-insured firm may be more than its reserves or financial capacity could bear if an unexpected case of AIDS or more than one catastrophic case was to develop during a plan year. For this reason, small groups, especially those which are self-insured, seek to spread the risks by obtaining reinsurance or "stop-loss" insurance.

This device is especially beneficial to small groups for which risks must be spread over a small number of employees. As the size of the group increases, the per capita risk decreases. Through reinsurance, the firm may agree to assume claims up to a given amount, then the reinsurance firm covers claims over that given amount. The firm may decide that it will cover up to 20 or 25 percent of the expected claims and have the reinsurance firm cover the remaining 75 to 80 percent of the claims.

The reinsurance mechanism enables the small group or firm to shift a major share of its own risks to a third party. It usually continues to be the primary focal point for administration of employees' claims, but it does not have to maintain as high a level of reserves to cover claims as it would had it not obtained reinsurance. It is also able to smooth out peaks and troughs of liability which could otherwise devastate the firms financial structure.

A target of reform in Congress has been the establishment of insurance pools in states so that small groups may obtain insurance at a reasonable price. Because a small number of AIDS cases or catastrophic/chronic cases in a small group may cause premiums to become out-of-reach, Congress has sought to set up insurance pools which:

1. Offer basic insurance at a low price due to economies of scale.
2. Provide small groups with a mechanism for spreading risks to a larger group.
3. Cover high-risk and high-cost groups which might not be able to obtain coverage otherwise.
4. Enable state and local governments to subsidize high-cost and high-risk groups as an incentive for businesses, which otherwise would not offer any kind of health care plan, to offer basic plans.

Part of the problem associated with the formation of such pools is the determination of how to spread the high-risk and high-cost cases among the members of the pool. Almost any system of assignment has both advantages and disadvantages both to the insurer and to the insured. The methods listed below have been considered by Congress and by underwriters as strategies for assignments to the reinsurance pools:

1. Proportionate allocation of high-cost and high-risk cases among pool members.
2. Random assignment of risks among pool members.
3. Share costs and allocate losses among pool members.
4. Have Insurance Commissioner decide on equitable method of allocation of risks and state subsidy of losses.

The first assignment method suggested above would have members of the reinsurance pool be assigned high-cost and high-risk cases based on the proportion of business that the reinsurer does in the state. The Commissioner would have worked out a method of assignment which would assign points to cases based on expected costs and/or risks and then would assign them to the participating members. Losses associated with the reinsurance pool would be reimbursed by the state on a proportional basis similar to the allocation of cases.

As is the case in high-risk automobile insurance in some states, high-cost and high-risk cases would be randomly assigned among the participating pool reinsurers. The random nature of assignment might cause short-term inequities or imbalances for some of the participating reinsurers, but over the long term, the system would be expected to produce an even distribution of high-risk and high-cost cases. If a given reinsurer should perceive that the system has dealt it an unfair share of undesirable cases, there is the possibility that it may retaliate against the undesirable cases with any number of punitive tactics, such as delayed claim processing or undue investigation of given claims or statements.

Perhaps one of the most equitable methods of allocation of high-cost and high-risk cases to participating reinsurance pool members would be to have reinsurers contribute funds against expected claims liabilities in proportion to the amount of business the reinsurer does in the state. At the end of the fiscal year, pool losses are allocated to reinsurers in proportion to the business they do in the state, or the state could reimburse the losses to the pool members according to their proportionate share of pool participation.

Where the reinsurance pool is set up in the state, the Insurance Commissioner will formulate a strategy for allocation of high-cost and high-risk cases among pool members, will calculate the expected case liability for the coming year, will design a reimbursement plan for any losses which are incurred by the pool members, and will formulate an incentive plan for insurer participation in the reinsurance pool. It is anticipated, however, that any national health care pool set up in the states will probably have mandatory participation by all insurers as a condition for doing business in the state.

Some target activities of reinsurance pools which have already been implemented in some states include:

1. Putting caps on the spread of rates between the lowest new business rates and the rates for existing similar coverage with similar case characteristics.
2. Creating uniformity in the limitations on preexisting conditions and/or completely eliminating them.
3. Guaranteeing renewability except as indicated in the language from the "Roybal Bill," H.R. 3535, which is model language for several of the House and Senate bills:

Grounds For Refusal To Issue Or Renew.—

(A) In General.—A carrier may refuse to issue or renew or terminate a plan only for—

(i) nonpayment of premiums,

(ii) fraud or misrepresentation, and

(iii) failure to meet minimum participation rates (consistent with subparagraph (B)).

(B) Minimum Participation Rates.—A carrier may require, with respect to an employer health plan, that a minimum percentage of full-time employees (who are not seasonal or temporary employees) eligible to enroll under the plan be enrolled, so long as such percentage is enforced uniformly for all employment groups of comparable size.[15]

4. Limits on the range of premium increases.

Polzer and Jones, in their National Health Policy Forum Issue Brief No. 596 describe the efforts to reform the small-group market in Connecticut's reinsurance pool. They indicate that the Connecticut system is somewhat a model in implementation of this type of reform package. They describe the system, in part, thusly:

Along with the rating and eligibility rules, Connecticut set up a reinsurance pool, administered by The Travelers. All insurers in the small-group health market are automatically members of the pool. Insurers can reinsure either individuals or groups through the pool, but must retain the first $5,000 of claims as their direct responsibility. For individuals, the reinsurance premium is 500 percent of a standard rate the pool establishes to cover expenses above $5,000 for people with similar characteristics and coverage. If the ceding carrier wishes to reinsure a group, the premium is 150 percent of a standard rate the pool establishes for groups with similar characteristics and coverage.[16]

UNDERWRITING RISKS—SOCIAL QUESTIONS

Legislators argue that insurers should "take all comers" because the insurance industry has typically been making their fair share of financial gains over the past few decades. They seem to feel that the insurers have a responsibility to provide insurance to all who need it. Their legislative efforts almost always contain elements of shifting the responsibility for high-cost and high-risk individuals and groups onto the insurers. This raises some interesting social questions regarding the assumption of risk in general.

In a competitive society, the incentive for assumption of risk is compensation. As the risk increases, the compensation for that risk increases. In the money market, a risky loan will call for a higher interest rate. Loans backed by the federal government generally yield much lower interest rates. In all segments of business, high risks are treated differently from low risks. Because health care is so vital to everyone, it is easy to lose the perspective that high-risk and high-cost groups and individuals are business risks. Whether the business wants to take those risks and what price tag is associated with those risks is a business decision. Politicians try to convince the public that such risks are a *responsibility* of the business, but the investors in the business (which usually do not include the government) may have other objectives *which do not include social welfare per se*.

Since the objective of insurers is to provide the best coverage at the lowest cost, where should the high-risk and high-cost individuals and groups fit into the picture? If reinsurance pooling is mandatory for high-risk and high-cost individuals and groups so that they may obtain insurance at a lower cost or even obtain it at all, should the government subsidize the assumption of risks beyond normal underwriting limits? How does the reinsurer price the reinsurance if groups and individuals have the option of remaining in or getting out of the pool? To what extent does mandatory reinsurance pooling create an incentive for non-participating insurers to exclude high-risk and high-cost individuals and groups from their plans? Should one expect one employer to subsidize the health care benefits of another employer?

The foundation of underwriting is that there are more or less autonomous, homogeneous categories of risks which should be rated differently from other more or less autonomous, homogeneous categories. In health care, the very young and the very old population categories have health care costs and risks that are several times those of other age categories. Males and females have different health care costs and different longevity. Professions which are largely sedentary have different health care risks and costs from those professions which are physically demanding and/or dangerous.

Since these different homogeneous categories have different risks and costs, and since actuarially determined rates are different for these categories, community rating—charging a single rate for those in a given community without regard to the category differences—would, at least, mean that:

1. Those who cost the most would not be paying what they are costing the community.
2. Those who cost the least would be subsidizing those who cost the most to the community.
3. Rates assigned to the community, if cutting across employers, may be inequitable to employer participants.
4. Community rates would not necessarily mean that the best coverage was enjoyed by the most people, that is, the allocation of health care resources may be inefficient in the aggregate.

The trend in the bills in the U.S. Senate and in the U.S. House of Representatives is toward elimination of most underwriting with respect to age, sex, condition of health, length of time enrolled, industry, or other risk characteristics. Despite the observation made in the earlier sections of this chapter that about 5 percent of the population incur about half of all medical expenses and that about 20 percent of the population incur about 80 percent of the medical costs, most bills in Congress which relate to national health care tend toward *community rating*. The language used is similar to the language in H.R. 3205, S. 1177, and H.R. 2535 (all identical wording) which state, in the language of the Rostenkowski bill, "Each such actuarial rate shall be uniform within each beneficiary class and *community*, and shall not vary among such individuals by age, sex, health, or other risk characteristics."[17]

In the next chapter, we look at the national health care concept of "play or pay," which has come to such prominence in legislative circles in the last two congresses. If the Congress wishes to implement the national health care system formally through the employer, this concept may provide a palatable alternative to a variety of mandated plans which may not be uniform across the states.

NOTES

1. Jerry S. Rosenbloom, *The Handbook of Employee Benefits: Design, Funding, and Administration* 2nd ed. (Homewood, Il.: Dow Jones-Irwin, 1988).
    2. *Ibid.*, especially chapter 44.

3. These conditions would normally be mentioned in "preexisting conditions" clauses in an *individual* health care policy and excluded, but in all of the universal coverage plans proposed and discussed later in this book they would be included in the plan, most of the time without even a waiting period. See the bills from Congress in chapters 5 through 7 of this book.

4. Most of the "preexisting conditions" clauses in plans "look back" to previous employment. If there was no claim in the last 3 months or no treatment in the last 6 months, then the employee will be covered. The usual waiting period for coverage under a new employer's plan is 3 to 6 months. That is the same period in some of the bills from Congress reviewed in this book.

5. Americans with Disabilities Act of 1990, Public Law 101–336 (Title I, S. 933, 101st Cong. and Title II, H.R. 2773, 101st Cong.) 101 Stat. 327, 26 July 1990.

6. Americans with Disabilities Act of 1990, *Ibid.*, Public Law 101–336 Sec. 102(c)(4)(A).

7. U.S. House of Representatives, "USHealth Program Act of 1991," H.R. 3535, 102d Cong., 2nd Sess. (Washington, D.C.: U.S. Government Printing Office, 1992).

8. U.S. House of Representatives, "Health Insurance Coverage and Cost Containment Act of 1991," H.R. 3205, 102d Cong., 1st Sess. (Washington, D.C.: U.S. Government Printing Office, 1991).

9. On an actuarial basis, they have a smaller basis for spreading any given risk. The percentage increase in the claims ratio for a given major claim will be greater than the same-sized claim from a larger entity.

10. Brian Harrigan and Nancy Jones, "The Cost Impact of AIDS on Employee Benefits Programs," *Compensation & Benefits Management* Vol. 3 (Winter 1987):27–29; Richard J. Donahue, "AIDS Cost Could Lead to National Health Insurance Plan," *National Underwriter* (9 Nov. 1987):6, 46; Donald L. Westerfield, "Analysis of Cost in Regulating and Treating AIDS and Related Diseases," *Proceedings of the 1988 Conference of the Business and Health Administration Association* (Mar. 1988):132–137.

11. U.S. House of Representatives, H.R. 2535 *Pepper Commission Health Care Access and Reform Act of 1991*, 102d Congress, 1st Session, 4 June 1991, pp. 75–76.

12. U.S. Senate, S. 1177, *Pepper Commission Health Care Access and Reform Act of 1991*, 102d Congress, 1st Session, 23 May 1991, p. 73.

13. U.S. House of Representatives, H.R. 3535 *USHealth Program Act of 1991*, 102d Congress, 1st Session, 9 October 1991, pp.142–143.

14. Karl Polzer and Judith Jones, "Risk Pools, Reinsurance, and Subsidies: Reforming the Small-Group Market for Health Insurance," Issue Brief No. 596, The George Washington University National Health Policy Forum, 1 June 1992, p. 4.

15. U.S. House of Representatives, H.R. 3535 *USHealth Program Act of 1991*, 102d Congress, 1st Session, 9 October 1991, p. 139.

16. Karl Polzer and Judith Jones, "Risk Pools, Reinsurance, and Subsidies: Reforming the Small-Group Market for Health Insurance," *op. cit.*, 5–6.

17. U.S. House of Representatives, H.R. 3205, *Health Insurance Coverage and Cost Containment Act of 1991*, 102d Congress, 1st Session, 2 August 1991, p. 81; U.S. House of Representatives, H.R. 2535, *op cit.*, p. 76; U.S. Senate, S. 1177, *op. cit.*, p. 73.

4

"Play or Pay" and Subsidies

The concept of "play or pay" revolves around the notion that all employers must provide a health care plan or pay a fee to a health care fund for a health care plan for each employee—*play* the health care game or *pay* a fee to have someone else play it for you. To contest the play or pay proposals that are being offered in Congress, Richard Armey of the Joint Economic Committee testified:

Play or pay proposals require employers to either purchase a basic package of health insurance benefits (play), or to enroll employees into a government-operated plan (pay) by paying a no-play tax or fine set at a predetermined percentage of each firm's payroll. While proposals vary, all would require employers to provide health insurance to workers who are employed for more than 18 hours a week. A 'simple' play or pay mandate costing 7 percent of a firm's payroll will cause over 710,000 workers to lose their jobs in the first year of implementation; 43 percent of all job losses, or 308,265 will occur in small businesses that employ fewer than 20 workers.[1]

It certainly seems reasonable enough to expect employers to provide their employees with health care coverage. As we analyze the play or pay concept from the business and social points of view, it may be well to keep in mind that *government and businesses have different responsibilities and objectives*. Governments are responsible for the health and welfare of their citizens. Businesses are responsible to their investors.

Businesses seek to provide the best possible product to the public at the lowest possible price while earning a reasonable return for its investors. Governments must provide a product to the public often at the highest possible price without regard to whether it earns a profit. Business and government responsibilities and objectives are different, clearly.[2]

How do we handle the situation where a small employer would like to provide health care benefits to its employees, but the cost of a health care plan is too expensive? The costs per employee are escalating at an alarming rate. Robert Patricelli, of the U.S. Chamber of Commerce, describes the burden of health care plans on the backs of small employers:

> Average employer health benefit costs are now running slightly over $3,000 per year . . . ; Family coverage alone is more than $4,500 per year. Adding $3,000 insurance plan to the salary of a $10,000 per year worker is a 30 percent compensation increase; for a worker earning $15,000 per year, it is a 20 percent increase. Given the precarious financial condition of a great many small businesses, imagine what an increase in mandated personnel costs of 20–30 percent would do. A study by the Partnership on Health Care and Employment estimates that between 630,000 and 3.5 million workers will likely lose their jobs under the type of mandate plans being advanced on Capitol Hill.[3]

Suppose the employer is in a very high risk business such as demolition by explosives, and all the employees are contracted. Should this employer be required to provide health care coverage to the contract employees? The mandated play or pay would mean that the employer would either provide coverage, even at phenomenal rates, or buy into the federally-sponsored plan.

MANDATED PLAY OR PAY

It is interesting to study the pattern of social welfare entitlements from the government and to note that an entitlement for even a short period takes the form of a *right*.[4] Health care in the workplace was originally a benefit which was the object of collective bargaining between management and a labor union. In earlier days, some labor unions were able to have health care plans included in the labor contract along with other benefits such as vacation days, sick days, life insurance, hourly rates, and others. In the mid- to late seventies and throughout the eighties, most employers which employed over 50 employees had been routinely including health care plans in the benefits packages of their employees.[5]

During the same time period, the federal government was systematically adding mandatory benefits for the employer to include in any benefits packages offered to the employees. Benefits such as:

• Pregnancy leave
• Mammograms
• Raising upper limit on retirement age
• COBRA coverage to extend health care coverage to separated employees and their dependents
• Accommodations to disabled employees[6]

and similar benefits appear to be in the public interest, but businesses argue that they are social welfare benefits and make no direct contribution to the productive capacity of the firm. Employers argue that such benefits should be the object of collective bargaining and should not be mandated by the government.[7]

The play or pay concept embodied in H.R. 3205, as introduced by Rep. Rostenkowski on August 2, 1991, is mandatory for those employers not already offering health care plans. The language of the bill is, in part, as follows:

Sec. 101. "Pay-Or-Play" Requirement.
(a) Premium Taxes.—(1) Subtitle C of the Internal Revenue Code of 1986 (relating to employment taxes) is amended by inserting after chapter 21 the following new chapter:
CHAPTER 21A—PUBLIC HEALTH PLAN TAXES
Sec. 3151. Imposition of Tax.
(a) Imposition of Tax.—In addition to other taxes, if an employee of any employer is not covered under a qualified employer health plan of such employer—
(1) Tax on Employers.—There is hereby imposed on such employer, with respect to having such employee in his employ, a tax equal to the employer rate percentage of the wages paid by such employer to such employee.
(2) Tax on Employees.—There is hereby imposed on the income of such employee a tax equal to the employee rate percentage of the wages received by such employee from such employer.
(b) Percentages.—For purposes of this section—

(1) Employer Rate Percentage.—The employer rate percentage for any calendar year is 80 percent of the percentage determined under paragraph (3) for such year.

(2) Employee Rate Percentage.—The employee rate percentage for any calendar year is 20 percent of the percentage determined under paragraph (3) for such year.

(3) Percentage Based On Public Health Plan Expenditures.—

(a) In General.—The percentage determined under this paragraph is—

(i) 9.0 percent for 1993, and

(ii) for any subsequent calendar year, the percentage determined by multiplying the update percentage for such year by the percentage determined under this paragraph for the preceding calendar year.[8]

Notice that the language of the Rostenkowski Bill above indicates that an employer will either provide a health care plan to its employees or will pay a excise tax. The language of Section 2100 of the same bill leaves no doubt about the mandatory nature of the plan:

Sec. 2100. Relation to "Pay-Or-Play" Requirement.

If an employer fails to enroll employees (and family members) under a qualified employer health plan in accordance with this title—

(1) the employer and employee are each liable for payment of an excise tax under section 3151(a) of the Internal Revenue Code of 1986, and

(2) the employer is required, under section 5000A of such Code, to provide information necessary to enroll such employees and family members under the public health plan under title XXII.[9]

There are a number of observations to be made from the language of the Rostenkowski Bill just cited. Probably the most important observation is that participation in the plan by employers and employees for an employer which does not provide a health care plan is mandatory. Both the employer and employee will make contributions to the plan—similar to the contributions to FICA as now implemented. One should note also that coverage of family members is mandatory—it is not possible for an employee to elect to take non-family coverage.[10]

REGRESSIVE RATE STRUCTURE

Section 3151 of the Rostenkowski Bill (H.R. 3205), as cited above, requires the imposition of a fixed percentage tax on employee wages received and on the employer wages paid. This fixed percentage, no matter what the percentage rate, will mean that low paid workers and low wage bill employers will contribute less to the plan in absolute dollars than will those higher paid workers and those employers with higher wage bills.[11] Additionally, it will mean that the relative weight of what is paid will be heavier for the workers and employers on the lower end of the scale. This is an example of a regressive tax—the burden of the tax is heavier for the low end of the wage and wage bill scale than for the high end of the scales. The Joint Economic Committee points out that:

> Mandated health care will eliminate over 710,000 jobs, throw those individuals in the weakest economic position out of work, force small entrepreneurs to close their doors and reduce the opportunity for low-wage workers to move to higher wage employment. Workers most likely to lose their jobs will be unskilled, less well educated, young, women or members of minority groups who currently have earnings at or near minimum wage.[12]

Up to this point, we have not addressed the role of special interest groups in shaping the national policy. Since health care is one of the most controversial social and political topics in the last decade, it would be reasonable to expect that groups like the American Association of Retired Persons (AARP) will immediately recognize the regressive nature of the employer and employee tax required by play or pay. It is expected that they will begin to offer a sliding scale of plan taxes which takes into account percentages of the national poverty level to reduce the burden on the low end of the wage scale.[13]

IMPLEMENTATION CONSIDERATIONS

If the objective of providing health care insurance at an affordable price to all in the plan is to be achieved, some problems will arise with regard to the tax placed on the workers and the employers:

1. It may be almost impossible for the government to forecast the extent of its liability without two or three years' experience.
2. It is unlikely that the tax will be sufficient to completely pay for the plan. A subsidy from the government will likely be necessary to make up plan losses.

3. If the plan rates are appreciably lower than the private plans, there surely will be a high rate of adverse selection. Sicker and older individuals and groups will select the government plan.

4. Employers typically paying low wages will almost surely choose the government plan rather than provide a plan of their own.

5. It is likely that the government-subsidized plan will cause private plans to shift their marketing and coverage toward the younger and healthier workers and groups, since the high-risk and high-cost workers and groups will opt for the lower priced government plan. The market may become dichotomized.

6. The subsidy for the government plan will become so politicized that the plan may become a national burden.

7. Subsidies may be spread unequally among the states, causing competition in congressional committees for health care funds for powerful states.

The list could go on and on, but it is sufficient to indicate that the pay or play concept seems reasonable and even simple on the surface, but that some of the social and political implications may be the ultimate road block to its implementation.

PUBLIC HEALTH TRUST FUND

Since tax dollars will be coming in to the U.S. Treasury from the taxes on the employees and from the employers to pay for the government sponsored plan, there must be some kind of trust set up within the government to administer those funds. One function of such a trust will be to estimate the amount of plan tax revenues and compare that against the estimated plan expenditures. Excesses and losses will have to be settled with the Treasury Department. H.R. 3205, the Rostenkowski Bill, provides for the creation of such a trust fund in the following section:

Sec. 2233. Public Health Trust Fund.—
(a) Establishment.—(1) In General.—There is hereby created on the books of the Treasury of the United States a trust fund to be known as the 'Public Health Trust Fund' (in this section referred to as the Trust Fund). The Trust Fund shall consist of such gifts and bequests as may be made as provided in paragraph (3) and such amounts as

may be deposited in, or appropriated to, such Trust Fund as provided in this part.

(2) Deposit of Taxes.—There are hereby appropriated to the Trust Fund amounts equivalent to 100 percent of the taxes imposed by—

(A) part VIII of subchapter A of chapter 1 of the Internal Revenue Code of 1986, and

(B) sections 3151, 5000A, and 5000B of such Code. The amounts appropriated by the preceding sentence shall be transferred from time to time from the general fund in the Treasury to the Trust Fund, such amounts to be determined on the basis of estimates by the Secretary of the Treasury of the taxes, paid to or deposited into the Treasury; and proper adjustments shall be made in amounts subsequently transferred to the extent prior estimates were in excess of or were less than the taxes specified in such sentence.[14]

One of the problems with the national health care system in the United Kingdom is the allocation of funds to the providers.[15] What seems to routinely happen is that the fund begins to get very low about August of each year. This calls for both rationing of funds to the providers and a rationing of health care services to the eligible subscribers throughout the rest of the year. As adjustments are made to even out the requirement for compensation for high-risk and high-cost cases, it is likely that powerful members of the congressional committees having oversight or control of the Trust Fund will be applying pressures to obtain greater proportions of funds for their districts to cope with the rationing problem.

An interesting anecdote, written by Anthony Schmitz in *In Health*, illustrates the very point made above. He describes an attempt by the state of Oregon to expand health care to its uninsured and the rationing problem it had to confront. He explained the situation as follows:

Hoping to get all its residents covered, Oregon recently passed legislation that will soon qualify 116,000 uninsured people for Medicaid, benefits they can't get now because they aren't poor enough. The state will then rank all medical procedures, weighing their costs against their known health benefits. Expensive, ineffective treatments will be lopped off the list. By this kind of rationing the state intends to save enough money to cover all the new people enrolled.

But a moral fog bank has now rolled in. The first attempt to create such a list ended in disaster, with care for thumb-sucking-related jaw problems ranked higher than some AIDS treatments. Even if they concoct an acceptable list, Oregon will have to ask Congress to let it rob Peter to pay Paul—trim the roster of treatments now available to Medicaid patients so it can offer the same reduced care to a larger group. The state should instead be raising taxes, critics say, and looking for ways to cut waste so everyone can be given decent care.

Among the states this is an increasingly common refrain: If we can't afford everything medicine has to offer, then how and where do we draw the line?[16]

The problems and their attempted solutions indicated in Schmitz's anecdote illustrate exactly the type of problems likely to be faced by the Trust Fund, especially since the fund will be experiencing a higher proportion of high-risk and high-cost cases—in effect an "insurer of last resort." Both implementation and administration problems already anticipated with such a mandatory system may be the greatest hurdle that Congress will have to overcome if it wants to adopt such a plan.

The advantages of the pay-or-play plan is that many small firms will opt to "buy in" to the plan and provide health care benefits to their employees since:

1. The plan will be compulsory.
2. The premiums will be more affordable than a comparable plan in the private market.
3. There will be relatively little administrative involvement in the plan by the employer.
4. Underwriting of high-risk and high-cost cases will be included in the plan coverage.
5. The plan is guaranteed renewable.

The major questions to be answered by both proponents of the pay-or-play concept and its opponents will be: "How many uninsured will have been covered by such a plan?" "Will the cost to the federal government be worth the benefit of the added workers and their families under the plan?" "What happens to the unemployed uninsured?" Other such questions will be nagging at the policymakers in Congress as this concept is debated in the national context.

In the next part of this book, we examine major laws and proposed legislation which have major impacts on the national health care question. It is surprising to the average person to learn that we actually do have a national health care system—it is not formalized and it is indirect. We will discuss this concept in the next part.

NOTES

1. Testimony of Richard Armey, Joint Economic Committee, before the U.S. House of Representatives, *Oversight Hearing on National Health Care Reform*, Serial No. 102–104, 7 May 1992 (Washington, D.C.: U.S. Government Printing Office, 1992), p. 1.

2. Testimony of Daniel Heslin, The ERISA Industry Committee, before the U.S. House of Representatives, *Oversight Hearing on National Health Care Reform, op. cit.,* pp. 60–70.

3. Testimony of Robert Patricelli before the U.S. House of Representatives, *Long-Term Strategies For Health Care*, Hearings Before the Committee on Ways and Means, House of Representatives, Serial 102–33, 102d Cong., 1st Sess., April 16–17, 23–25, 1991 (Washington, D.C.: U.S. Government Printing Office, 1992), p. 558.

4. Kenneth Buchi and Bruce Landesman, ''Health Care in a National Health Program: A Fundamental Right'' in Robert Huefner and Margaret Battin, eds., *Changing to National Health Care: Ethical and Policy Issues* (Salt Lake City, Utah: University of Utah Press, 1992), pp. 191–208; Allen Buchanan, ''Competition, Charity, and the Right to Health Care'' in Thomas Attig et al., eds., *The Restraint of Liberty* (Bowling Green, Ohio: Bowling Green State University, 1985):129–143.

5. Testimony of Dallas Salisbury before the U.S. House of Representatives, *Long-Term Strategies For Health Care, op. cit.,* pp. 264–280.

6. Donald Westerfield, *Mandated Health Care: Issues and Strategies* (New York: Praeger, 1991); G. J. Minc, ''Providing A Section 129 Dependent Care Assistance Program Through A Section 125 Cafeteria Plan,'' *Taxes* (May 1988):361–367; ''Public And Private Issues In Financing Health Care For Children,'' *ERBI Issue Brief* (June 1989):1–15.

7. Jack Bresch and Frederick Krebs, ''Compulsory Employee Benefits: Pro And Con,'' *Association Management* (April 1989):86–91; Susan J. Daley, ''The Meaning Of Mandated Health Benefits,'' *Corporate Health* (July/Aug. 1988):12–15; L. Dosier and L. Hamilton, ''Social Responsibility and Your Employer,'' *Personnel Administrator* (Apr. 1989):88, 90, 92, 95; ''Employers Would Cut Wages, Benefits, If Minimum Health Care Bill Becomes Law,'' *Benefits Today* (6 Nov. 1987):384.

8. U.S. House of Representatives, *Health Insurance Coverage and Cost Containment Act of 1991*, H.R. 3205, 102d Congress, 1st Session, 2 August 1991 (Washington, D.C.: U.S. Government Printing Office, 1991), pp. 6–7.

9. U.S. House of Representatives, *Health Insurance Coverage and Cost Containment Act of 1991*, H.R. 3205, *op. cit.,* p. 17.

10. Notice that the wording ''(and family members)'' is always inserted after the word ''employees'' throughout Title XXI—Requirement For Enrollment of Employees Under a Qualified Employer Health Plan in *Health Insurance Coverage and Cost Containment Act of 1991*, H.R. 3205, *op. cit., passim.*

11. Testimony of John Motley, III, before the U.S. House of Representatives, *Long-Term Strategies For Health Care, op. cit.,* 596–613.

12. Testimony of Richard Armey, Joint Economic Committee, before the U.S. House of Representatives, *Oversight Hearing on National Health Care Reform, op. cit.*, p. 28.

13. Most of the "reform" plans discussed in subsequent chapters of this book have incorporated the "sliding scale" of premiums based on percentages of the poverty level.

14. U.S. House of Representatives, H.R. 3205, *op. cit.*, pp. 84–85.

15. John Lister, "Proposals for Reform of the British National Health Service," *New England Journal of Medicine* (30 March 1989):877–880; Stephen Birch, "DRGs U.K. Style: A Comparison of U.K. and U.S. Policies for Hospital Cost Containment and their Implications for Health Status," *Health Policy* 10:2(1988):143–154; Theodor Litman and Leonard Robins, *Health Politics and Policy* 2nd ed., (New York: Delmar Publishers, 1991); Christopher Ham, *Health Policy in Britain: The Politics and Organization of the National Health Service* (London: Macmillan, 1985).

16. Anthony Schmitz, "Taking Cover in Ohio, New York, and Oregon," *In Health* (January/February 1991):41.

Part II

Health Care Proposals in Congress

5

Major "Universal" Plans in Congress

It is hard to imagine that when Theodore Roosevelt was running against Woodrow Wilson for president of the United States in 1912, Roosevelt endorsed the Progressive Party platform that pledged to provide the American people with some form of insurance to protect themselves against the hazards of sickness. By the 1930s, when Franklin Delano Roosevelt came into office, the American people, having just experienced The Great Depression, were able to obtain a whole array of social programs including Social Security, Federal Deposit Insurance Corporation (FDIC) insurance, unemployment insurance, and a number of welfare programs at the local and state levels of government.[1]

By the time Harry Truman became president in 1945, American's opinions about social welfare programs had galvanized into organized and formal resistance to any form of "socialism." This wall of resistance was faced by Truman when he introduced a bill of rights for Americans which included the right of all Americans to adequate protection from the economic consequences of sickness. Remarkably, as mentioned in the previous chapter, the American Medical Association fought Truman's proposal "tooth-and-nail," calling it a socialist reform measure. This attitude prevailed until the mid-1960s, when the tactic of focusing attention on insurance for the elderly proved to be successful.[2]

President Lyndon Johnson came in with a sweeping mandate to make changes in the social welfare system. By mid-1964 to early 1965 the idea of Medicare and Medicaid became palatable enough to both Republicans and Democrats that the Medicare-Medicaid package was enacted and implemented as universal health care coverage for the aged.[3] Since that time, Americans have been more receptive to the notion that the health care system must have a program that contains comprehensive care, include as much of the population as possible (be "universal" in coverage), and must have the support of both federal and state governments.

We see the change in the attitudes from the Harry Truman era to the present in the structure and scope of the legislation presented in this chapter.

Six major universal health care plans were introduced into Congress during the 102d Congress:

1. "The Medicare Universal Coverage Expansion Act of 1991," H.R. 1777, sponsored by Sam Gibbons (D.-FL).
2. The "Universal Health Care Act of 1991," H.R. 1300, sponsored by Marty Russo (D.-IL) et al.
3. "Health USA Act of 1991," S. 1446, sponsored by Robert Kerrey (D.-NE).
4. The "Comprehensive Health Care for All Americans Act," H.R. 8, sponsored by Mary Rose Oakar (D.-OH) et al.
5. "Health Care Cost Containment and Reform Act of 1992," H.R. 5502, sponsored by Pete Stark (D.-CA).
6. The "National Health Insurance Act," H.R. 16, sponsored by John Dingel (D.-MI) et al.

What all six bills have in common is the type of language that makes the provision of health care in America truly universal—that is, very few, if any, exceptions to access. Additionally, these plans do not look to the employer as a major participant as administrator, facilitator, or subsidizer of the health care system. Of the six bills mentioned, none really spell out in detail what the costs will be nor who will bear the ultimate financial burden of the program.

THE MEDICARE UNIVERSAL COVERAGE EXPANSION ACT, H.R. 1777—GIBBONS

Representative Gibbons's plan, H.R. 1777, is the simplest stated plan, but is more explicit and comprehensive than all the others. Just three typewritten pages, the plan outlines a strategy for universal coverage through a single payer, single administration system. Sections 1 and 2 of his description of the bill are as follows:

> Section 1: Short title (vis., the "Medicare Universal Coverage Expansion Act of 1991").
> Section 2: (a) Amends section 226 of the Social Security Act ("SSA") to provide for entitlement to benefits under parts A and B of the medicare program for all citizens, permanent residents, and lawful permanent aliens in the United States. This effectively provides medicare coverage for all Americans.
> (b) Conforming amendment to medicare part B to clarify that everyone entitled to benefits under medicare part A is also entitled to benefits under part B.
> (c) Amends section 1862 of SSA to eliminate a provision that makes medicare payments secondary to those of employers in certain cases. This assures that medicare will be the first payor for health care for all individuals, rather than being secondary to employer health plans.
> (d) Repeals various sections of SSA, relating to eligibility for medicare benefits, no longer needed as a result of the expansion of medicare eligibility to cover the entire population.[4]

Notice here that this bill would place the entire national health care system under a revised and expanded Medicare system. It does not preclude other insurance programs from providing benefits, but *all* Americans would be covered under the plan regardless of age.

UNIVERSAL HEALTH CARE ACT, H.R. 1300—RUSSO

The "Universal Health Care Act of 1991," H.R. 1300, was sponsored by Representative Marty Russo (D.-IL) and others on March 6, April 23, August 26, and November 6, 1992 and then on January 22 and February 24, 1992. This bill is closely related to those of Senator Kerrey and Representative Oakar, with the exception that Russo's bill is a federally administered program. Russo's plan would be administered through the Administrator of the Health Care Financing Administration (HCFA) and financed through a National Health Trust Fund.[5]

A description of the major features of Russo's bill is outlined in his testimony before the House Committee on Ways and Means.[6] In that testimony, Russo indicates that the major provisions of the plan are:

1. Universal access to health care through a single, publicly-administered program.
2. Comprehensive benefits for all Americans, including hospital and physician care, dental services, long-term care, prescription drugs, mental health services, and preventive care.
3. Freedom of choice so that everyone can choose their own physician or source of care.
4. Cost savings through annual budgets and a national fee schedule so that health dollars are spent efficiently and effectively.
5. Progressive financing to make health care affordable for all.
6. Quality measures to improve the type of medical care we receive.
7. Uniform federal standards to guarantee that all Americans receive full access to comprehensive, quality care coupled with state administration so that implementation decisions reflect local needs.[7]

The Department of Health and Human Services (DHHS) would have responsibility for administering the program at the national level, but the states could, with the approval of the DHHS, agree to take responsibility for the program at the state level.

"The program would be financed through a new 6% payroll tax on employers, an increase in the corporate income tax from 34% to 38% for businesses with more than $75,000 in profits, increases in the personal income tax from 15%-28%-34% with a top rate at 38% for families with incomes over $200,000, reforms of the tax code, a long term care/health premium equal to the Part B premium plus $25/month for the elderly above 120% of poverty, an increase in the amount of Social Security benefits included as taxable income from 50% to 85%, state payments equal to 85% state Medicaid effort plus an annual per capita fee of $85, and federal contributions equal to current spending on health care. All revenues collected for health care would be placed into a National Health Trust Fund and could only be used for health care expenses."[8]

This plan would have the unique feature of providing American citizens with "identical benefits from the health care provider of their choice." It is this sentence that makes Russo's plan sound like that of Representative Sam Gibbons. Indeed, the two plans are almost identical with respect to benefits and administration.

HEALTH USA ACT, S. 1446—KERREY

Senator Robert Kerrey (D.-NE), introduced his "Health USA Act of 1991," S. 1446, to the U.S. Senate Committee on Finance on July 11, 1991, as a bill "to provide for an equitable and universal national health care program administered by the States. . . . "[9] The language of this bill, S. 1446, and that of Representative Oakar's H.R. 8 is almost identical throughout, except that Representative Oakar's bill has additional sections, namely,

1. Division B—Life Care Long-Term Care Protection Act
2. Division C—Grants to States for Establishment and Implementation of State Health Objectives Plans
3. Division D—Independence for Older Americans.

With those exceptions, both bills have *identical titles and subtitles*. The most shocking sections of both the Kerrey and Oakar bills are the sections outlining "no competition" with services provided by the state plans. For example, in Kerrey's S.1446, page 19, Section 201, and page 25, Section 202, we read, respectively:

(d) NO DUPLICATE PRIVATE INSURANCE.—Private insurance for health care services may be sold in a State only for services not covered under the State program of such State
(j) NO DUPLICATE PRIVATE INSURANCE.—Private insurance for long-term care services may be sold in a State only for services not covered under the State program of such State.[10]

Other features of the Kerrey plan include annual deductibles of $100 for each individual and $300 for a family consisting of more than 2 individuals, copayment of $5 to be charged and collected at the first physician visit for an illness, and cost sharing limits of:

1. $1,000 per family of 1 individual
2. $1,500 per family of 2 individuals
3. $2,000 per family of more than 2 individuals
4. No cost sharing for basic services or inpatient care.[11]

To administer the national health care program under the Kerrey plan, a National Health Care Commission would be set up under the Department of Health and Human Services. This Commission would be responsible for overall administration of the provisions of the Act and would be responsible for developing guidelines for the state programs.

Probably the most important section in the Kerrey plan to employers, the self-employed, and to individuals regarding the burden of financing the plan is Section 331, outlining the payroll taxes, employer excise taxes, and changes in the structure of the federal income tax for individuals. If one had to predict where this plan will hit a "snag" in Congress, it would be in this section dealing with the taxes. It is interesting to compare the provisions in this bill with the simplicity of the Gibbons bill (H.R. 1777) already discussed. While the burden of taxes may be comparable in both bills, the explicit language in Kerrey's bill seems to be much more of a "bitter pill" than that of the Gibbons bill.

COMPREHENSIVE HEALTH CARE FOR ALL AMERICANS ACT, H.R. 8—OAKAR

Representative Mary Rose Oakar (D.-OH) introduced the "Comprehensive Health Care for all Americans Act," also called the "Claude Pepper Comprehensive Health Care Act," jointly to the Committees on Ways and Means and Energy and Commerce of the U.S. House of Representatives on January 3, 1991. As mentioned in the discussion of the Kerrey bill above, the wording of many sections of her bill and Kerrey's are identical. An example of such wording is observed in Sec. 101(a) under the title of Universal Eligibility:

(a) IN GENERAL.—Each individual who is a resident of the United States and is a citizen or national of the United States or lawful resident alien (as defined in subsection (c)) is eligible to enroll with a qualified health plan for coverage for health benefit under this division under the State CHC [comprehensive health care] program in the State in which the individual maintains a primary residence.[12]

In testimony before the Committee on Ways and Means of the U.S. House of Representatives, Representative Oakar outlined the most important features of her program.[13] Many of the basic services are standard throughout almost all of the plans, including her own, but Representative Oakar specifically listed the following major plan features:

1. Preventive health care in all areas.
2. Acute and outpatient care.
3. Long-term care, including home- and community-based care, homemaker services, heavy chore service, home health care services, respite care services and nursing home benefits up to 6 months.
4. Cancer screening, vaccinations, etc.
5. Research to find cures for diseases.
6. Let the various nonprofit organizations and insurance companies, if they wanted to, bid [on providing the state services] . . . so that each State would have the opportunity to put that high standard out for anyone who wanted to get into the system, just as we do for Federal employment and you and I . . . might be able to choose from three or four types of coverage.[14]

As mentioned earlier about the Kerrey plan, Representative Oakar's plan also has the "no duplicate private insurance" clause in Section 201(d) that covers both basic health care services and long-term care services provided by the states. What this will mean for the insurance companies operating throughout the states and just how they will interpret this section will temper their support of this bill or the Kerrey bill.

The extra subsections of the Oakar plan deal mainly with spelling out some of the specific details of the services not explicitly mentioned in Kerrey's bill. Additionally, the Oakar plan would set up a National Comprehensive Health Care Board which would not only be responsible for the overall administration of the plan but would also be responsible for developing guidelines for the various states so that they could implement the program. Each state would have a State Comprehensive Health Care Board to administer the state programs.

Under Subtitle C—Sources of Revenues, the bill addresses the issue of how the program will be financed in the various states. It states that:

Each state shall be responsible for establishing a financing program for implementation of the State CHC program in the State. Such financing program may include State funding from general revenues, earmarked taxes, sales taxes, subject to section 332, employer and employee health insurance premiums and cost-sharing, and such other measures consistent with this division as the State may provide.[15]

This differs from Senator Kerrey's plan somewhat in the respect that the Kerrey plan looks to various payroll taxes, employer excise taxes, and a revision in the income tax structure. Oakar's bill leaves it to the state to decide which taxes are more appropriate to finance the program.

HEALTH CARE COST CONTAINMENT AND REFORM ACT OF 1992, H.R. 5502—STARK

To understand the Health Care Cost Containment and Reform Act of 1992 (H.R. 5502), one must go back to 1991 and review the MediPlan Act of 1991, H.R. 650 by Representative Fortney (Pete) Stark.[16] One of the characteristics of the Stark (H.R. 5502) bill that makes it so different from the other universal coverage bills is the inclusion of a "means test." When he testified before the U.S. House Committee on Ways and Means, he testified, "My bill has three principle tenets . . . every resident in the United States ought to have medical care available as a matter of right. Second, every provider of this medical care has, as a matter of right, an expectation of reasonable compensation. [Third] Every person in America pays for that care according to their ability to pay."[17]

Both the MediPlan bill and the Health Care Cost Containment and Reform Act of 1992 bill would be supported by a two percent tax on gross income, as well as tax-exempt income, deferred income and other forms of income not explicitly identified now, but will be by the secretary of the plan. The revenues from all the tax sources will be paid into the MediPlan Trust Fund. Additionally, under MediPlan, both the employer and employee pay premiums. The employer pays up to $800 per year per worker (80% of the Mediplan premium) and the employee pays premiums and taxes on a sliding scale—the remaining $200 per year per person (20% of the Mediplan premium) for those with incomes above the poverty line.[18]

Under MediPlan, benefits for children, pregnant women, and low-income persons are provided without payment of premium. Families with incomes above twice the poverty level will pay an additional tax of two percent on all income, as mentioned above. This supplemental two percent tax becomes effective on income above $32,000.[19]

Under the Health Care Cost Containment and Reform Act of 1992, H.R. 5502, there are linkages between the Secretary of Health and Human Services and the 50 states and the District of Columbia for maintaining plan consistency and payment continuity. The plan would ensure all the benefits of the MediPlan through the existing Medicare and Medicaid structure—Titles XVII and XIX of the Social Security Act. Claims, payments, patient data, and provider data would be stored and transferred through an electronic data network which would be designed, implemented, and maintained through the

1. Workgroup on Electronic Data Interchange
2. National Uniform Billing Committee
3. Uniform Claim Task Force
4. Computer-based Patient Record Institute
5. American National Standards Institute.

For the purpose of providing services throughout the United States through such an electronic network, the plan calls for the establishment of "claims clearinghouses." Section 223 of H.R. 5502 states:

For purposes of carrying out this section, the Secretary shall designate within the continental United States areas encompassing approximately 5 million residents each. To the extent practicable, the areas shall be reasonably contiguous with State boundaries. Each area, and each of the States of Alaska and Hawaii, is referred to in this section as a "clearinghouse area."[20]

Similar to the systems in the United Kingdom and in Canada, where individuals are assigned to a center associated with their residence, this plan assigns each individual and each provider to a Health Claims Clearinghouse (electronic data network). These clearinghouses will verify eligibility for benefits and will track patients' benefits and records through the electronic interchange of records and through the use of an individual identity card. Section 223(c) states, in part:

ASSIGNMENT OF RESIDENTS AND PROVIDERS TO HEALTH CLAIMS CLEARINGHOUSES.—For purposes of carrying out this section—(1) RESIDENTS.—Each individual—
(A) who is a medicare beneficiary or is entitled to benefits under a health benefit plan with an agreement with a clearinghouse, and
(B) has a principal residence in a geographic area, shall be assigned to the clearinghouse for that area.
(2) PROVIDERS.—Each health service provider shall be assigned to the clearinghouse for the area in which the provider is located to provide services.[21]

The above outlined electronic network is unique to the national health care plans presented to Congress to date. Other features of the bill which are similar to the other universal health care bills are open enrollment, guaranteed renewability of coverage, community rating, and payments using the resource-based relative value scale (RBRVS) for physician and other professional medical services.[22]

While the combination of H.R. 650 and H.R. 5502 is probably the most comprehensive and carefully laid out plan for universal health care, its very detail and the massive changes involved may make it vulnerable to attack from those proposing simpler "bandaid" approaches.

NATIONAL HEALTH INSURANCE ACT, H.R. 16— DINGELL

Representative John Dingell (D.-MI) introduced his "National Health Insurance Act," H.R. 16, to the Committees on Energy and Commerce and Ways and Means on January 3, 1991. Like previously discussed plans, the Dingell plan establishes a National Health Care Trust Fund to administer funds throughout the states. State implementation of the plan is spelled out in Section 4 of the Findings and Declaration of Purpose: "Sec. 4. In carrying out these policies, it is the intention of Congress that the major administrative responsibilities be placed in the hands of local bodies representing both those who pay for and receive services and those who render services, and operating within the framework of plans made by the several States . . . "[23]

The architecture of the plan is different from the others, due in part to the way the states will design and implement their approved plans and in the way that the benefits through Medicare will be coordinated. Section 701 of the plan suggests that the benefits under Medicare may not be the same benefits as non-Medicare plan benefits.

The most unique feature of the Dingell plan is the establishment of a "value added tax" similar to that in the United Kingdom. This tax is outlined in Title X—Value Added Tax and National Health Care Trust Fund. Provision for this tax is accomplished by inserting "Chapter 30— Value Added Tax" before Chapter 31 of Subtitle D of the Internal Revenue Code of 1986. Section 3901 of Chapter 30 states: "Sec. 3901. IMPOSITION OF TAX. (a) GENERAL RULE.—A tax is hereby imposed on each taxable transaction. (b) AMOUNT OF TAX.—Except as otherwise provided in this chapter, the amount of the tax shall be 5 percent of the taxable amount."[24]

Much of the rest of Chapter 30 discusses those transactions or categories of transactions which are subject to the 5 percent value added tax. It might be pointed out here that many health care analysts have argued that a value added tax would be the simplest method of paying for a universal health care plan. The opposing argument is that such a tax is regressive and will be a heavier burden on the poor than some other tax that is related to income with a floor, below which tax is not paid. The Stark plan would be such an example of that kind of income tax with a sliding scale of tax liability.

COMPARISON OF PLANS

Perhaps the most important question raised by the plans presented in this chapter is whether the voters in America are willing to have comprehensive health care for *all* citizens, without qualification, or whether they want to incrementally ease into some sort of national health care structure. This question is not posed trivially.

The universal health plans are, for the most part, really universal, that is, they really seek to include both the employed and the unemployed in their structure. There are a number of arguments regarding whether there will be some savings in the universal plans which will offset the really mind-boggling expenditures required to implement such programs. Additionally, there is the major obstacle of deciding what kind of premium or taxing mechanism can both be equitable and approach budget neutrality. We will analyze these arguments in chapter 12 when we consider the national debate on how the national dollar should be allocated among competing national objectives.

NOTES

1. Rashi Fein, "Prescription for Change," *Modern Maturity* (August-September 1992):22–35.

2. Frank Campion, *The AMA and U.S. Health Policy: Since 1940* (Chicago: Chicago Review Press, 1984); Lawrence D. Brown, "Introduction To A Decade Of Transition," *Journal Of Health Politics, Policy And Law* 16 (1986):569–570.

3. Karen Davis and Cathy Schoen, *Health and the War on Poverty: A Ten-Year Appraisal* (Washington, D.C.: The Brookings Institution, 1978); David Callahan, *Setting Limits: Medical Goals In An Aging Society* (New York: Touchstone/Simon & Schuster, 1987); Madelon Finkel and Hirsch Ruchlin, *Retiree Health Care: A Ticking Time Bomb* (Brookfield, Mass.: International Foundation of Employee Benefit Plans, 1988).

4. U.S. House of Representatives, "Medicare Universal Coverage Expansion Act of 1991," H.R. 1777, 102d Cong., 1st Sess., *Congressional Record—Extension of Remarks*

(16 April 1991):E1261-E1262; see also his mimeo "Section-By-Section Description of H.R. 1777, The Medicare Universal Coverage Expansion Act of 1991," dated 4 June 1991 in personal communication to the author.

5. See Sections 2131 and 2133 of U.S. House of Representatives, "Universal Health Care Act of 1991," H.R. 1300, 102d Cong., 2nd Sess. (Washington, D.C.: U.S. Government Printing Office, 1992).

6. U.S. House of Representatives, *Long-Term Strategies For Health Care*, Hearings Before the Committee on Ways and Means, House of Representatives, Serial 102–33, 102d Cong., 1st Sess., April 16–17, 23–25, 1991 (Washington, D.C.: U.S. Government Printing Office, 1992), pp. 492–505.

7. *Ibid.*, p. 494.

8. *Ibid.*, p. 501.

9. U.S. Senate, "Health USA Act of 1991," S. 1446, 102d Cong., 1st Sess. (Washington, D.C.: U.S. Government Printing Office, 1991), p. 1.

10. U.S. Senate, "Health USA Act of 1991," S. 1446, *op. cit.*, Title II—Benefits and Providers, Sec. 201(d), p. 19, and Sec. 202(j), p. 25.

11. *Ibid.*, pp. 64–65, Sec. 333(b).

12. U.S. House of Representatives, "Comprehensive Health Care for All Americans Act" (Claude Pepper Comprehensive Health Care Act), H.R. 8, 102d Cong., 1st Sess. (Washington, D.C.: U.S. Government Printing Office, 1991), p. 5.

13. U.S. House of Representatives, *Long-Term Strategies, op. cit.*, pp. 515–524.

14. *Ibid.*, pp. 517–518.

15. *Ibid.*, pp. 34–35.

16. U.S. House of Representatives, "Health Care Cost Containment and Reform Act of 1992," H.R. 5502, 102d Cong., 2d Sess. (Washington, D.C.: U.S. Government Printing Office, 1992) and "MediPlan Act of 1991," H.R. 650, 102d Cong., 1st Sess. (Washington, D.C.: U.S. Government Printing Office, 1991).

17. U.S. House of Representatives, *Long-Term Strategies, op. cit.*, pp. 479–480.

18. *Ibid.*, pp. 483–484.

19. See the plan description in U.S. House of Representatives, *Long-Term Strategies, op. cit.*, pp. 485–487.

20. U.S. House of Representatives, "Health Care Cost Containment and Reform Act of 1992," H.R. 5502, 102d Cong., 2d Sess. (Washington, D.C.: U.S. Government Printing Office, 1992), Sec. 223, p. 95.

21. *Ibid.*, Sec. 223(c)(1)-(2), pp. 97–98.

22. See the Press Release #1A from the Subcommittee on Health, Committee on Ways and Means, dated July 7, 1992.

23. U.S. House of Representatives, "National Health Insurance Act," H.R. 16, 102d Cong., 1st Sess. (Washington, D.C.: U.S. Government Printing Office, 1991), Sec. 4, p. 5.

24. *Ibid.*, Sec. 3901(a)-(b), p. 68.

6

"Pay-or-Play" Proposals in Congress

We discussed the concept of the "pay-or-play" plans and the notion of employers and given categories of employees having to subsidize other employers and other categories of employees, especially under the community rating mandate. On the surface, it would seem reasonable to expect all employers would be willing to offer some sort of basic health care packages to their workers, especially if the premiums were uniform across large categories of employers, if the plans were guaranteed renewable, and if it were mandatory for at least some insurers to provide the basic health care plan to all employers.

Those who propose the mandatory "pay-or-play" health care plans base their arguments for employers adopting such plans on some existing facts observed in federal and state regulations related to employee benefits. It is a fact that the federal and state governments already regulate at least some portion of employee benefits, irrespective of the size of the employer. It is a fact that about 62.5% of the uninsured and underinsured are part-time or full-time workers. There is a popular, but as yet unproven, argument that a happy worker is a productive worker, and, presumably, if workers receive more benefits they are happier and more productive.

PEPPER COMMISSION PROPOSALS— ROCKEFELLER, WAXMAN

Before formally discussing the actual Pepper Commission proposals by Senator John Rockefeller and Representative Henry Waxman, it is

appropriate to mention the tribute that Representative Mary Oakar made
to Senator and Representative Claude Pepper in her H.R. 8, referred to
both as the "Comprehensive Health Care for All Americans Act" and
the "Claude Pepper Comprehensive Health Care Act," introduced to the
House joint Committee on Ways and Means and Energy and Commerce
on January 3, 1991, and by others on March 6, 1991, and September
24, 1991. Section 2 of the bill states: "Sec. 2 Honoring Claude Pepper.
The comprehensive health care program provided under this Act is enacted
in honor of Senator Claude Pepper and his 50 years of public service
efforts to provide comprehensive health care and long-term care for Americans of all ages."[1]

Two bills, based on the work of the Pepper Commission—U.S. Bipartisan Commission on Comprehensive Health Care—were introduced,
first, in the U.S. Senate by Senator John Rockefeller, S. 1177, *Pepper
Commission Health Care Access and Reform Act of 1991* on May 23,
1991,[2] and, second, in the U.S. House of Representatives by Representative Henry Waxman, H.R. 2535, *Pepper Commission Health Care
Access and Reform Act of 1991* on June 4, 1991.[3] They resemble the
"play-or-pay" plans proposed by Representative Rostenkowski (especially H.R. 3205), discussed in an earlier chapter, in the respect that the
employer is expected to enroll employees in "a qualified employer health
plan (or in the public health insurance plan, if elected by the employer
under Section 2105)."[4]

In testimony before the Committee on Ways and Means, U.S. House
of Representatives,[5] Senator John Rockefeller IV, Chairman of the Pepper
Commission, outlined the blueprint for national health care proposed by
the Pepper Commission:

1. First all workers must be entitled to health care coverage in
   their jobs. . . . After a brief period for adjustment, the Commission would require these employers (with more than 100
   workers) to cover employees and their nonworking dependents.
2. The Commission therefore recommended small group insurance reform that would guarantee open enrollment, community rating and access to a federally-defined minimum standard
   of benefits—reforms aimed to make coverage *available* to
   small groups. Under our proposal, tax credits would also be
   provided to small employers, to reduce their insurance costs.
3. Rather than simply *requiring* any employer to buy private

coverage, whatever its costs, the Commission would therefore give employers a choice: purchase private coverage or purchase coverage from a newly-established public program at subsidized prices.

4. We therefore recommended replacing Medicaid with a new federal program that would provide the same minimum standard of benefits that employers would have to provide. The public program would pay providers rates based on Medicare rules, in place of Medicaid's abysmally low rates.

5. The Commission would achieve these objectives [cost containment and quality] through a number of actions, including: a basic benefit package that emphasizes managed care and other innovative delivery mechanisms; extension of Medicare's increasingly effective methods of provider payment to the new public program; and data collection, outcomes research, and practice guidelines to help public and private payers alike use their dollars wisely.[6]

When Representative Bill Archer of Texas asked Senator Rockefeller what kind of taxes would have to be raised in order to implement the provisions of the Pepper Plan, Senator Rockefeller replied:

... they go all the way from a 1.9 percent increase—I am just taking the highest dollar figure in each of the options—a 1.9 percent increase in the FICA rate, a 4 percent value-added tax with exemptions for food, shelter, health, that is another big one; 33 percent top rate for income tax, 7 percent surtax, that is another option; supplemental tax of 4.5 percent on modified gross income over $32,000 for joint returns. That last one would raise $75 billion. This the entire Pepper Commission recommendations I am talking about, not just the $24 billion but the $70 billion needed for the whole Pepper Commission plan, which includes long-term care.[7]

The Rockefeller plan, S. 1177, "Pepper Commission Health Care Access and Reform Act of 1991," contains eight major titles.

Title I—Access To Private Or Public Health Insurance For Basic Health Services Through Employment. This title of the bill addresses the treatment of full-time, part-time, and seasonal workers as well as family members and dependents of those who are employed in any manner.

Title II—Access To Health Insurance For Basic Health Services Through A

Public Health Insurance Plan.   This title primarily discusses the treatment of persons who are not employed, who have low incomes, and those who need assistance in paying premiums. It also outlines the benefits, deductibles, coinsurance, stop-loss insurance, and specifications of the Public Health Insurance Trust Fund. It is the major title of the bill with Parts A through H.

Title III—Quality Assurance And Cost Containment.   Title III deals mainly with the mechanics of cost containment with some discussion of quality of care.

Title IV—Group Health Insurance Reform.   This is the most technical part of the plan, dealing with stringent enforcement provisions, preexisting conditions, definitions of qualified plans, reinsurance plans, managed care, insurance providers, community rating, and definitions of benefits.

Title V—Expansion Of Primary Care And Public Health Delivery Capacity In Meeting Health Objectives.   Title V mainly deals with funding, reports, and studies associated with public health. The reference to ''Healthy People, 2000'' is a reference to a follow-up study to be periodically reported to the Secretary of Health and Human Services on the state of the nation's health.

Title VI—Financing And Tax-Related Provisions.   While this title of the bill addresses funding and taxes to fund the plan, the most outstanding section of this title is Section 606, which repeals the COBRA continuation requirement. The discontinuance is a phased-in process, depending on the size of the employer group—ranging from the fourth year after the plan implementation for large employers to the sixth year after the plan implementation for very small employers.

Title VII—Medicare And Medicaid Amendments.   The major focus of this final title is a reform of Part B of Medicare and of the Medicaid program. There is a ''coordination of benefits''-type arrangement with the national health plan to ensure that the coverage will be broad enough to cover those covered now and the target unemployed and low-incomed families and individuals.

Title VIII—Conforming Changes To ERISA.   This title explicitly repeals Part 6 of subtitle B of title I of the Employee Retirement Income Security Act of 1974 (ERISA), also known as the COBRA portion of ERISA. The COBRA part of ERISA has been aggressively fought by businesses of all sizes as an anti-competitive, cost-shifting measure passed by Congress in response to pressures by pressure groups which would not have to pay for COBRA's mandate.

The Waxman plan, H.R. 2535, "Pepper Commission Health Care Access and Reform Act of 1991," is almost identical in language to the Rockefeller plan, since they were both designed for the same purpose. When Representative Henry Waxman testified before the *Long-Term Strategies For Health Care* hearings, Waxman described his bill as follows:

> My bill will build an employer-based system for health care coverage for working people and their dependents. The Kennedy-Waxman bill, last year, would have achieved this result through a mandate on employers to provide coverage. In the legislation I intend to introduce next month, I have adopted the pay-or-play model recommended by the Pepper Commission.
>
> It will also include a residual public program to assure access to basic benefits for those not enrolled in private plans. I intend to include in the bill cost containment policies modeled on those developed in this committee and my own, for Medicare.
>
> In addition, my bill would put in place reforms in insurance marketing and rating practices that will be particularly important to small businesses. With respect to this last point, I do want to emphasize that insurance reforms, alone, will not move us toward our goals. Let's not kid ourselves. If we eliminate medical underwriting in private insurance and require community rating of policies and we do not set standards for basic benefits, or require employers to provide coverage, the result, I fear, will be more uninsured persons.
>
> Community rating and open enrollment can only succeed when the costs of health care are spread across the full population of an area. Otherwise, the insured risk pool will have adverse selection and premiums will soon be unaffordable.[8]

The "pay-or-play" provisions of S. 1177 and H.R. 2535 were designed so that costs for the national health care system are "shifted" to the employer for those who are employed. The "community rating" provisions of both bills cause costs for the health plans for the unhealthy to be paid for or "subsidized" by those who are healthy. Both bills contain *identical language* regarding both underwriting for individuals (actuarial determination of rates charged) and community rating (guaranteeing issue regardless of health status, medical histories, claims experience, or lack of insurability) for groups:

Actuarial Rates: Each such actuarial rate shall be uniform within each beneficiary class, benefit package, and community, and shall not vary among such individuals by age, sex, health, or other risk characteristics.[9]

Community Rating: Subject to the succeeding provisions of this subsection, a carrier that offers a health plan (including a reinsurance plan, but only if offered to a self-insured employment-related health plan) to small employers located in a community must offer the same plan to any other small employer located in the community.[10]

While the "pay-or-play" concept has already been discussed in a previous chapter, the impact on business and its prospects for passage through Congress will be discussed at length in a subsequent chapter. On its face, the concept looks like it could be implemented easily, since much of the insurance-provider-payer infrastructure has been laid by other federal and state mandates.[11]

The Rockefeller and Waxman plans spelled out the role of employers in the "pay-or-play" scheme. The three plans to be discussed below differ somewhat from the Pepper Commission plans. Nevertheless, they are also of the "pay-or-play" variety. The three plans to be spotlighted are the "USHealth Program Act of 1991," H.R. 3535—Roybal,[12] "HealthAmerica: Affordable Health Care for All Americans Act," S. 1227—Mitchell,[13] and the "Comprehensive Health Insurance Plan of 1991 (CHIP)," S. 2114—Packwood.[14]

USHEALTH PROGRAM ACT, H.R. 3535—ROYBAL

Representative Edward Roybal (D.-CA) introduced the "USHealth Program Act of 1991," H.R. 3535, to the U.S. House of Representatives Committees on Ways and Means, Energy and Commerce, and Education and Labor on October 9, 1991. The plan is essentially a pay-or-play plan that contains basic health care and long-term care, with other insurance and tax reforms related to health care. The plan explicitly spells out its objectives for employer participation in Section 2101(a)(1): "Except as provided in this part, each employer shall, in accordance with this title, enroll each of its . . . employees . . . in a qualified employer health plan (or in the USHealth Program, if elected by the employer under section 2105)."[15]

Notice that the employer has two options available, either provide the employer's own plan or pay for the USHealth Program. Under Section

2102 of the plan, the employer must either enroll part-time employees in the USHealth Program or pay a premium to the USHealth Program Trust Fund. Employers must even make premium payments for seasonal and temporary employees under the provisions of Section 2103, if they are not enrolled in an employer qualified health care plan.

The Roybal plan additionally requires that employer plans have an "open door" to all persons, irrespective of "health status, claims experience, receipt of health care, medical history, or lack of evidence of insurability of an individual."[16] What this means is that there will be no underwriting considerations when considering applicants to the employer plan. The plan further explicitly directs that the actuarial determination of rates be "community rating" as outlined in Section 601(a)(2)(B): "Each such actuarial rate shall be uniform within each beneficiary class and community, and shall not vary among such individuals by age, sex, health, or other risk characteristics."[17]

The rationale for requiring employers to provide insurance of their own or to enroll employees in the USHealth Program is that a large proportion of the uninsured are actually employed, as discussed in a previous portion of this book. What this type plan actually accomplishes is a shifting of social responsibilities for health care from the federal and state governments to the employer.

In testimony before the U.S. House of Representatives Committee on Ways and Means, Representative Roybal outlined some of the financing and employer participation in his plan. He states:

Under "USHealth" states would be required to maintain their current level of spending on health care and beneficiaries would pay some premiums, coinsurance, and deductibles. Individuals and families with incomes below 100% of the poverty level would not have to pay anything; those with incomes between 100% and 200% would pay on a sliding scale. Medicaid would be eliminated.

"USHealth" has not been costed-out yet, but the Pepper Commission estimated that a plan of this type could be provided for about $66.6 billion in new federal spending: $24 billion to cover the uninsured; $18.8 billion to cover care in a nursing home; and $24 billion to pay for care in the home.

"USHealth" could be financed largely by lifting the cap on wages subject to the health insurance and social security taxes (essentially taxing income above $53,400). The roughly 5% of Americans earning more than $53,400 a year would join other workers in paying the 7.65% payroll tax on their full income.[18]

HEALTHAMERICA: AFFORDABLE HEALTH CARE FOR ALL AMERICANS ACT, S. 1227—MITCHELL

On June 5, 1991, Senator George Mitchell (D.-ME), introduced his "HealthAmerica: Affordable Health Care for All Americans Act," S. 1227, to the U.S. Senate. While the Roybal plan was a bit more subtle regarding the "pay-or-play" consequences of the USHealth Program, the language of the Mitchell bill is quite explicit. The first provision of the bill under Title XXVII—Basic Health Benefits for Employees and Their Families, Section 2701(a)(1) states:

IN GENERAL.—Except as provided in part B, each employer shall—

(A) enroll each of its employees (other than part-time employees) and their families in a health benefit plan in accordance with part B; or
(B) make a contribution under title V of the HealthAmerica Act, for the coverage for such employees and their families under the public health insurance plan established under title XXI of the Social Security Act.[19]

Some of the features of the plan include preemption of state mandated health care benefits, reform of small group insurance, tax deductions for plans for small-and medium-sized businesses, and standards for the promotion of managed care. Probably the most impressive characteristic of the Mitchell plan is its preoccupation with regulations. The benefits are outlined in the plan in adequate detail, but most of the document is involved in intricate discussions of regulations associated with taxes, alternative plans, advisory committees, and authorizations and certifications. In short, the document (S. 1227) seems to be less a health care plan than a set of unnecessarily burdensome regulations on business.

COMPREHENSIVE HEALTH INSURANCE PLAN (CHIP), S. 2114—PACKWOOD

Senator Bob Packwood (R.-OR), on November 26, 1991, introduced his bill entitled "Comprehensive Health Insurance Plan of 1991 (CHIP)," S. 2114, to the U.S. Senate Committee on Finance.[20] Like the bills previously discussed in this section, Packwood's bill is a "pay-or-play" bill which mandates that employers provide certain plans or face rather severe tax consequences. What makes the Packwood plan unique is the requirement to offer employees a range of alternative plans—the "play" concept—or face punitive tax liabilities—the "pay" concept.

Notice how different the language of the Packwood bill is regarding the employer's obligation to offer different types of health care plans:

(a) GENERAL RULE.—Except as provided in succeeding subsections of this section, each employer shall, in accordance with this part, offer to each of its eligible employees a qualified employer plan. Such offer—

(1) shall include at least—

(A) 1 basic health plan, and

(B) 1 basic coordinated care plan (if the employer is located in the service area of such a plan), and

(2) may include 1 or more—

(A) enhanced health plans, or

(B) enhanced coordinated care plans.[21]

The above language spells out the mandatory "play" section of the bill, even though there are descriptions of the plans and constraints on the implementation and administration of the plans throughout the bill. The penalty or "pay" part of the bill is found in Section 102. Tax Penalties on Noncomplying Employers and Insurers. Chapter 43 of the Internal Revenue Code of 1986 is amended to include Sec. 4980C, Failure to Offer to Enroll Eligible Employees in Qualified Employer Plans. Sections (a) and (b)(1) of Sec. 4980C are given below:

(a) GENERAL RULE.—There is hereby imposed a tax on the failure of any person to offer to enroll any eligible employee in a qualified employer plan under part A of title XXI of the Social Security Act.

(b) AMOUNT OF TAX.—

(1) IN GENERAL.—The amount of the tax imposed by subsection (a) on any failure with respect to an eligible employee shall be $50 for each day in the noncompliance period with respect to such failure.[22]

The Packwood plan is applicable to employees working at least 25 hours per week and at least 16 weeks per year. It may also include consultants and contractors if the Secretary "determines that the consulting arrangement or contract was entered into to avoid the requirements of this title."[23]

The "pay-or-play" plans require employers to bear a continued burden for the health care of their employees *and their dependents*. This raises a social welfare question about the conflict of objectives to produce a quality product at the lowest possible price with a fair return to investors for their risks and the inclusion in the price of that product social costs mandated on them by the federal and state governments. Scholars, business leaders, members of Congress, and health policy analysts are increasingly raising the question of *whether the employers should be in the health care business at all*.

NOTES

1. U.S. House of Representatives, "Comprehensive Health Care for All Americans Act" (Claude Pepper Comprehensive Health Care Act), H.R. 8, 102d Cong., 1st Sess., 1991, p. 2.

2. U.S. Senate, "Pepper Commission Health Care Access and Reform Act of 1991," S. 1177, 102d Cong., 1st Sess. (Washington, D.C.: U.S. Government Printing Office, 1991).

3. U.S. House of Representatives, "Pepper Commission Health Care Access and Reform Act of 1991," H.R. 2535, 102d Cong., 1st Sess. (Washington, D.C.: U.S. Government Printing Office, 1991).

4. U.S. House of Representatives, "Pepper Commission Health Care Access and Reform Act of 1991" H.R. 2535, 102d Cong., 1st. Sess., 1991, p. 7.

5. U.S. House of Representatives, *Long-Term Strategies For Health Care*, Hearings Before the Committee on Ways and Means, House of Representatives, Serial 102–33, 102d Cong., 1st Sess., April 16–17, 23–25, 1991 (Washington, D.C.: U.S. Government Printing Office, 1992), p. 379. The whole statement by Senator Rockefeller is given at pp. 374–403.

6. U.S. House of Representatives, *Long-Term Strategies, op. cit.*, p. 379.

7. *Ibid.*, pp. 383–384.

8. U.S. House of Representatives, *Long-Term Strategies, op. cit.*, p. 511. The text of his statement is given at pp. 510–515.

9. See p. 73 in S. 1177 and p. 76 in H.R. 2535.

10. See p. 177 in S. 1177 and p. 185 in H.R. 2535.

11. See arguments in chapters 8, 9, and 13 of Donald Westerfield, *Mandated Health Care: Issues and Strategies* (New York: Praeger, 1991) and U.S. House of Representatives, "Medicare Universal Coverage Expansion Act of 1991," H.R. 1777, 102d Cong., 1st Sess., *Congressional Record—Extension of Remarks* (16 April 1991):E1261-E1262; see also his mimeo "Section-By-Section Description of H.R. 1777, The Medicare Universal Coverage Expansion Act of 1991," dated 4 June 1991 in personal communication to the author.

12. U.S. House of Representatives, "USHealth Program Act of 1991," H.R. 3535, 102d Cong., 2nd Sess. (Washington, D.C.: U.S. Government Printing Office, 1991).

13. U.S. Senate, "HealthAmerica: Affordable Health Care for All Americans Act,"

S. 1227, 102d Cong., 1st Sess. (Washington, D.C.: U.S. Government Printing Office, 1991).

14. U.S. Senate, "Comprehensive Health Insurance Plan of 1991 (CHIP of 1991)," S. 2114, 102d Cong., 1st Sess. (Washington, D.C.: U.S. Government Printing Office, 1991).

15. U.S. House of Representatives, "USHealth Program Act of 1991," H.R. 3535, *op. cit.*, Sec. 2101(a)(1).

16. U.S. House of Representatives, "USHealth Program Act of 1991," H.R. 3535, *op. cit.*, Section 2710(a).

17. *Ibid.*, Sec. 601(a)(2)(B), p. 321.

18. U.S. House of Representatives, *Long-Term Strategies, op. cit.*, p. 373.

19. U.S. Senate, "HealthAmerica: Affordable Health Care for All Americans Act," S. 1227, 102d Cong., 1st Sess. (Washington, D.C.: U.S. Government Printing Office, 1991), pp. 4–9.

20. U.S. Senate, "Comprehensive Health Insurance Plan of 1991 (CHIP of 1991)," S. 2114, 102d Cong., 1st Sess. (Washington, D.C.: U.S. Government Printing Office, 1991).

21. *Ibid.*, Sec. 2101(a).

22. *Ibid.*, Sec. 4980C(a),(b)(1).

23. *Ibid.*, Sec. 2103(b)(2).

7

Health Care Reform Proposals in Congress

The health care proposals reflected in the congressional bills discussed in the previous chapter were designed primarily as comprehensive health care packages with reform as a secondary purpose. The proposals that we examine in this chapter are primarily health care market reform measures which try to also expand coverage through the small group markets. These are more "incremental" in their approach to the solution of the health care crisis and have been criticized, whether with justification or not, as "bandaid" approaches. Just how many of the now uninsured would benefit from these measures is an open question. The American Medical Association (AMA) feels strongly, however, that insurance market reform is an absolutely necessary first step to obtaining system-wide reform. James S. Todd, Executive Vice President of the AMA states:

> Before small employers can be expected to provide health coverage, small group insurance must be made affordable and accessible. The following reforms are essential:

- Community rating across all small groups;
- No pre-existing condition limitations;
- Guaranteed acceptance of all employees, possibly through an assigned-risk approach, with an initial minimum coverage period of two years;
- Guaranteed renewability with limits on premium increases; and
- The required offering by carriers of an essential benefits health policy.[1]

Employers could argue that there are some cost-shifting and conflict of interest statements implications within the AMA reform proposals, especially in the light of the fact that they will not have to bear the major financial burden of their recommendations and that they will stand to gain financially through increased utilization of their health care facilities and physicians. Despite these arguments, there are some important considerations within the AMA reform proposals that we will see in most of the reform measures now in Congress that are discussed in this chapter.

The way we will analyze the proposals presented in this chapter is to look at clusters of proposals that either use almost identical language or that seek almost identical reform measures. Those proposals presented are the major ones being considered in Congress to date. Their order of discussion below has no relationship to the importance of the reforms they seek to accomplish.

"CORE BENEFIT" PLANS

Three bills have almost identical language and section numbers, and have almost identical reform objectives. Two of the bills, H.R. 2121 and S. 700, are almost identical in every respect. S. 2036 contains all the sections of H.R. 2121 and S. 700, but is a bit more comprehensive and has a much broader scope. The three bills are formally:

1. "Health Insurance Reform Act of 1991," H.R. 2121, introduced by Representative Fortney "Pete" Stark (D.-CA)[2]
2. "American Health Security Act of 1991," S. 700, introduced by Senator David Durenberger (R.-MN)[3]
3. "Access to Health Care for All Americans Act of 1991," S. 2036, introduced by Senator Robert Kasten (R.-WI)[4]

Generally, all three bills seek to have employees guaranteed minimum "core" benefits which roughly coincide with those provided under title XVIII of the Social Security Act, Parts A and B. In S. 700 and S. 2063, both bills have identical language which outline a "Medplan" and "core" benefits:[5]

(d) MEDPLAN.—For the purposes of this section—
(1) CORE MEDPLAN.—The term 'core Medplan' means an accident and health plan which provides the core benefits described in paragraph (3).

(2) STANDARD MEDPLAN.—The term 'standard Medplan' means an accident and health plan which provides—
(A) the core benefits described in (3), and
(B) the supplemental benefits described in paragraph (4).

The language of H.R. 2121 varies slightly from the language given above for that section. All three plans have subsections which provide for guaranteed eligibility, guaranteed renewability, limitations on coverage of preexisting conditions, "index" rating, and small employer coverage. S. 2036 includes sections of reform of medical malpractice, rural health care, community health centers, and provisions for long-term care.

Section 5000a—Failure to Satisfy Certain Standards for Health Insurance, is identical for all three bills. This section outlines the tax imposed by the Secretary of Health and Human Services on persons who fail to meet both the issuance requirements of 5000B and contractual requirements of 5000C of the respective plans. All three plans include an amendment to chapter 47 of the Internal Revenue Code of 1986 to include "Chapter 47—Certain Group Health Plans" "Subchapter A—Nonconforming Group Health Plans."[6] Typically the nonconforming groups could be small employer purchasing groups, self-insured plans, or qualified health maintenance organizations (HMOs).

HEALTH EQUITY AND ACCESS IMPROVEMENT ACT

Senator John Chafee (R.-RI) proposed the "Health Equity and Access Improvement Act of 1991," S. 1936, to the Committee on Finance on November 7, 1991.[7] His bill contains almost all of the provisions in Representative Rod Chandler's (R.-WA) bill, "Small Employer Health Insurance Incentive Act of 1991," H.R. 2453, except that Chandler's bill goes more into the details of preemption from state insurance mandates for qualified small employer purchasing groups than does that of Chafee.[8] Senator Chafee's Section 221 on Qualified Small Employer Purchasing Groups is also more comprehensive than Representative Chandler's Section 3 on the same subject.[9]

Probably the most interesting feature of the Chafee bill is Title IV—Public Health Provisions, Subtitle A—New Basic Health Care Program, Sec. 401—Establishment of Basicare Program.[10] The Basicare service is established in this bill "For the purpose of providing basic health care benefits to low-income uninsured individuals not eligible for coverage under title XIX of this Act . . . '' This is complemented with grants to provide service to ''medically underserved individuals'' and ''medically underserved areas.'' The funds for these projects involve federal-state matching funds to ''need-adjusted'' populations.

STATE UNIVERSAL HEALTH CARE

Improvements to the HealthAmerica Act, S. 1669—
Simon

The ''Improvements to the HealthAmerica Act of 1991,'' S. 1669, introduced to the U.S. Senate Committee on Finance by Senator Paul Simon (D.-IL) is a four-barreled shot at national health care.[11] Title I— Cost Containment, Subtitle A—Federal Health Expenditure Board sets up a new title under the Public Health Service Act—Title XXVII— Basic Health Benefits for Employees and Their Families. The duties of this board are to develop a national health care plan and a way to implement it. Subtitle B—State Purchasing Consortia set up the framework for a State Consortium with membership stated as ''All providers and purchasers of health insurance and health care in the State, including business, labor, and consumer organizations, shall be eligible to become members of the consortium in such State.''[12]

These consortia will set quality standards for state health care plans, will ''convene negotiations with health care providers and purchasers,'' and will generally act as a large health care cooperative.

The third prong of this plan really gets to the meat of a state health care plan called ''AmeriCare.'' Title II—State Single Payer Option sets forth the following authorization: '' . . . a State may establish a universal health care system for the residents of such State, to be supported by revenues generated from State tax assessments, if such system provides universal health care coverage for all residents of the State that is at least as comprehensive as the health care coverage required under this Act and Amendments made by this Act.''[13]

This is really the ''meat'' of Senator Simon's bill. It then authorizes federal matching funds to help fund such a program. Notice, however, that such plans are left to the state to design, implement, and maintain. The state program will be under the authority of the Federal Health Expenditure Board established earlier in the Act.

The fourth feature in the Simon bill covers early retirees, strikers, and individuals whose employers' businesses have failed.[14] This would establish benefits provided under expanded availability of Medicare for those persons over 60 after the third year of the program and benefits under AmeriCare for others eligible under this title.

National Health Care and Cost Containment Act, H.R. 2530—Sanders

The "National Health Care and Cost Containment Act," H.R. 2530, was introduced to the U.S. House of Representatives Committees on Energy and Commerce and Ways and Means on June 4, 1991, by Representative Bernard Sanders (I.-VT).[15] The Sanders plan calls for federal block grants to states that provide insured health services under a state health care insurance plan. The block grant would cover the uninsured, underinsured, long-term care, and out- of-pocket expenses in any state plan. The bill then provides for:

1. Comprehensiveness of benefits—Sec. 203.
2. Universality of coverage—Sec. 204.
3. Portability of benefits—Sec. 205.
4. Accessibility to benefits—Sec. 206.

Compared to most of the other plans, the Sanders plan is a "universal" plan for states. The fixed block grants from the Health Care Financing Administration would be a matter to be worked out both with respect to equity among the states and relative need.

OTHER COMPREHENSIVE REFORM PLANS

There are three U.S. Senate bills which have titles which would lead one to expect perhaps some sort of universal coverage. While the number of persons who may actually benefit may be quite large, they, nevertheless, are actually just reforms for specific target populations. They are presented below in more or less a rank order according to the size of the target populations they are expected to affect.

Comprehensive American Health Care Act, S. 454—McConnell

Senator Mitch McConnell (R.-KY) introduced the "Comprehensive American Health Care Act," S. 454, to the U.S. Senate Committee on Fi-

Table 7.1
Long-Term Care Insurance Tax Credit

If Adjusted Gross Income is:	Percentage Is
Less than $25,000	70%
$25,000 but less than $30,000	50%
$30,000 but less than $35,000	30%
$35,000 but less than $40,000	10%
$40,000 or more	0%

nance on February 21, 1991.[16] The essence of this bill is its provision for federal tax credit for "qualified health insurance expenses" for those who are not covered by an employer plan. Exceptions are those individuals who receive benefits under part A of title XVIII of the Social Security Act.

The remaining portion of Title I of the McConnell bill deals with standardizing rural health care payments. Title II lays out a proposal for medical malpractice reform and to establish reasonable availability and affordability of liability insurance. Perhaps one of the strongest sections of his bill is Title III, which covers long-term care insurance and plans. The long-term insurance tax credit feature is a sliding scale as shown in Table 7.1.

What Table 7.1 shows is the percentage of qualified long-term care premiums paid during a given taxable year that may be applied as a credit against an individual's tax liability for that tax year. A similar sliding scale is given for the dollar amount deductible for individuals with attained age before the close of the taxable year.

Subtitle B of the McConnell bill amends Section 1832(a) of the Social Security Act to extend Medicare benefits to several specialized categories of individuals, including in-home respite care, home care for intravenous drug therapy, and extended home health services.

Comprehensive Health Care Act, S. 314—Cohen

The "Comprehensive Health Care Act of 1991," S. 314, introduced by Senator William Cohen (R.-ME), contains a section addressing separate average standardized amounts for hospitals in rural areas similar to that of the McConnell bill.[17] More than anything else, the bill seeks to reform health care claims procedures through consultations between the National Association of Insurance Commissioners and parties providing health care services and health care insurance.

Other reform objectives of the Cohen bill are to make health insurance more affordable for self-employed individuals, give tax incentives for physicians practicing in rural areas, and provide more lenient tax treatment for long-term care insurance provided by employers.

Unique features of Senator Cohen's bill are the provisions for what would normally be called the "catastrophic care" cases. They are treated in:

1. Sec. 705, Exclusion from Gross Income for Amounts Withdrawn from Individual Retirement Plans for Qualified Long-Term Care Insurance Premiums
2. Sec. 706, Tax Treatment of Accelerated Death Benefits Under Life Insurance Contracts
3. Sec. 707, Tax Treatment of Companies Issuing Qualified Terminal Illness or Dread Disease Riders
4. Title VIII—State Uninsurable Pool Programs.

These sections typically are not found in other health care reforms and provide special relief to areas that involve amounts of an individual's income that are often devastating. The state uninsurable pool concept is implemented in several states, but most of the "universal" coverage plans would have the so-called "open door" provisions that would vitiate the necessity to establish such pools.

Better Access to Affordable Health Care Act, S. 1872—Bentsen

Senator Lloyd Bentsen (D.-TX) introduced his "Better Access to Affordable Health Care Act of 1991," S. 1872 to the U.S. Senate Committee on Finance on October 24, 1991.[18] It is a companion bill to Representative Daniel Rostenkowski's "Health Insurance Reform and Cost Control Act of 1991," H.R. 3626.[19] The Bentsen bill provides, under Title I of the bill, for a 100 percent federal income tax deduction for health insurance costs to small employers. It also establishes support for small employer health insurance purchasing programs. Probably the major features of the Bentsen bill are the provisions for portability of health care benefits, outlined in Title III, and the expansion of Medicare benefits outlined in Title V.

Some of the group insurance reforms mentioned in the Bentsen bill are:

1. Guaranteed availability of health insurance to small employers
2. Guaranteed renewable insurance for small employers
3. Guaranteed eligibility for all individuals in a group
4. Limits on preexisting conditions
5. Limits on the variabililty of premiums among similar groups with respect to health status, claims history, occupation, industry, and other risk factors.

As indicated above, the Bentsen plan and the Rostenkowski plan are quite similar in purpose and reform measures, especially those outlined above and the requirement for insurers to offer at least two types of group coverage, which may include a very basic health care plan or a more comprehensive standard health care plan.

State Health Reform Opportunity Act, H.R. 2297— Markey

Representative Edward Markey (D.-MA) introduced the "State Health Reform Opportunity Act of 1991," H.R. 2297, to the U.S. House of Representatives Committees on Energy and Commerce and Ways and Means on May 9, 1991.[20] The purpose of the bill is outlined in Sec. 2(a), which states, "The Secretary of Health and Human Services shall provide grants of up to $1,000,000 to each State to assist the State in developing and implementing a health care process that provides for the participation described in subsection (b) and that will result in development of a single, unified health care plan designed to accomplish the goals specified in subsection (c)."

At first glance, the above portion of the bill seems like the $1 million per state is a "drop in the bucket" compared to what such a plan may cost. Section 3 of the plan, however, really drops a bomb with its provisions to "transfer to state of federal health care expenditures under the Medicare, Medicaid, and other federal programs for services covered under the state health care plan." That is a remarkable transfer of responsibility from federal programs to state authority—title XVIII of the Social Security Act, title XIX of the Social Security Act, title V of the Social Security Act, and other programs at the discretion of the Secretary of Health and Human Services.

If states choose to accept the responsibility of a universal state plan, the Markey plan (just 5 pages in length) would affect one of the most sweeping changes of all the reform plans. The $1,000,000 "seed money" may not be enough to entice the states to make such a drastic change in the structure of their health care systems.

SPECIALIZED REFORM PLANS

In this final section, we consider two specialized health care reform packages, both from the U.S. Senate. The bills are described below in order of the scope of their coverage.

Medicaid Glideslope Act, S. 1211—Graham

Except for the short title section, which is Section 1, the "Medicaid Glideslope Act of 1991," S. 1211, introduced to the U.S. Senate Committee on Finance by Senator Bob Graham (D.-FL), there is only one other section, Section 2. The title of Section 2 tells just exactly what this whole reform plan is about: "Sec. 2. Optional Expansion of Medicaid Coverage to Individuals with Family Incomes Not Exceeding 300 Percent of the Income Official Poverty Level." How the "Glideslope" got into the title, only the Lord knows! Perhaps one could imagine the glideslope as a sliding scale of premiums and cost sharing as outlined in Sec.2(d).

This 7-page bill, if implemented by the states, will cover a large number of uninsured and underinsured workers and their dependents. It is this segment of the population who are most at risk, and this segment of the population would cover those individuals with moderate incomes as indicated in Table 7.2. The 1989 poverty thresholds were reported by the U.S. Bureau of the Census.[23]

Notice from the table that a four person family could be making $34,986 dollars per year and still qualify for the expanded Medicaid coverage under the Medicaid Glideslope Act as proposed by Graham. This could be thought of as a fairly comprehensive health care "safety net" for the millions of workers with marginal jobs.

Health Care Access and Affordability Act, S. 1995—Specter

The final reform proposal to be considered in this chapter is the "Health Care Access and Affordability Act of 1991," S. 1995, introduced to the U.S. Senate Committee on Labor and Human Resources by Senator Arlen

Table 7.2
1989 Poverty Levels at Three Times the Given Poverty Levels

1.	1 Person - $5,807	X 300% =	$17,421
2.	2 Persons - $7,431	X 300% =	$22,293
3.	3 Persons - $9,095	X 300% =	$27,285
4.	4 Persons - $11,662	X 300% =	$34,986
5.	5 Persons - $13,792	X 300% =	$41,376

Specter (R.-PA).[24] This is a somewhat narrow reform proposal, despite the implied scope of its title, which amends the Public Health Service Act to include revised health care services for:

1. Tuberculosis prevention
2. Lead Poisoning prevention
3. Sexually transmitted diseases
4. Migrant health centers
5. Community health centers
6. Services for the homeless
7. Substance abuse programs
8. Breast and cervical cancer prevention

The plan also contains cost containment proposals of the type proposed by other plans. While this is not exactly a comprehensive health care plan, it does explicitly address some of the areas of health care concern which have been most prominent in the public eye through news specials on television and in the print media.

NOTES

1. James Todd, Statement before the U.S. House of Representatives, *Long-Term Strategies For Health Care* Hearings Before the Committee on Ways and Means, House of Representatives, Serial 102–33, 102d Cong., 1st Sess., April 16–17, 23–25, 1991 (Washington, D.C.: U.S. Government Printing Office, 1992), pp. 780–781.

2. U.S. House of Representatives, "Health Insurance Reform Act of 1991," H.R. 2121, 102d Cong., 1st Sess. (Washington, D.C.: U.S. Government Printing Office, 1991).

3. U.S. Senate, "American Health Security Act of 1991," S. 700, 102d Cong., 1st Sess. (Washington, D.C.: U.S. Government Printing Office, 1991).

4. U.S. Senate, "Access to Health Care for All Americans Act of 1991," S. 2036, 102d Cong., 1st Sess. (Washington, D.C.: U.S. Government Printing Office, 1991).

5. See Sec. 5000B(d)(1)-(2) of both U.S. Senate, "American Health Security Act of 1991," S. 700, and "Access to Health Care for All Americans Act of 1991," S. 2036.

6. See Sections 5000E(b) of S. 700 and S. 2036 and Section 5000D(b) of H.R. 2121.

7. U.S. Senate, "Health Equity and Access Improvement Act of 1991," S. 1936, 102d Cong., 1st Sess. (Washington, D.C.: U.S. Government Printing Office, 1991).

8. See Section 2 of U.S. House of Representatives, "Small Employer Health Insurance Incentive Act Of 1991," H.R. 2453, 102d Cong., 1st Sess. (Washington, D.C.: U.S. Government Printing Office, 1991) versus Section 222 of U.S. Senate, "Health Equity and Access Improvement Act of 1991," S. 1936.

9. See S. 1936, Sec. 221 versus H.R. 2453, Sec. 3, both cited in the previous note.

10. U.S. Senate, "Health Equity and Access Improvement Act of 1991," S. 1936, op. cit., pp. 100–105.

11. U.S. Senate, "Improvements to the HealthAmerica Act of 1991," S. 1669, 102d Cong., 1st Sess. (Washington, D.C.: U.S. Government Printing Office, 1991).

12. U.S. Senate, "Improvements to the HealthAmerica Act of 1991," S. 1669, op. cit., Sec. 2721(b)(2).

13. Ibid., Title II—State Single Payer Option, p. 83.

14. See Title III—Coverage of Early Retirees, Strikers and Individuals Whose Employers' Businesses Have Failed, Sec. 301, of S. 1669, cited in the previous note.

15. U.S. House of Representatives, "National Health Care and Cost Containment Act," H.R. 2530, 102d Cong., 1st Sess. (Washington, D.C.: U.S. Government Printing Office, 1991).

16. U.S. Senate, "Comprehensive American Health Care Act," S. 454, 102d Cong., 1st Sess. (Washington, D.C.: U.S. Government Printing Office, 1991).

17. U.S. Senate, "Comprehensive Health Care Act of 1991," S. 314, 102d Cong., 1st Sess. (Washington, D.C.: U.S. Government Printing Office, 1991). For a comparison of the sections dealing with rural hospitals see Subtitle B of S. 454 and Title I of S. 314.

18. U.S. Senate, "Better Access to Affordable Health Care Act of 1991," S. 1872, 102d Cong., 1st Sess. (Washington, D.C.: U.S. Government Printing Office, 1991).

19. U.S. House of Representatives, "Health Insurance Reform and Cost Control Act of 1991," H.R. 3626, 102d Cong., 2nd Sess. (Washington, D.C.: U.S. Government Printing Office, 1992).

20. U.S. House of Representatives, "State Health Reform Opportunity Act of 1991," H.R. 2297, 102d Cong., 1st Sess. (Washington, D.C.: U.S. Government Printing Office, 1991).

21. U.S. Senate, "Medicaid Glideslope Act of 1991," S. 1211, 102d Cong., 1st Sess. (Washington, D.C.: U.S. Government Printing Office, 1991).

22. U.S. Senate, "Health Care Access and Affordability Act of 1991," S. 1995, 102d Cong., 1st Sess. (Washington, D.C.: U.S. Government Printing Office, 1991).

23. U.S. Department of Commerce, *Statistical Abstract of the United States 1991* (Washington, D.C.: Bureau of the Census, 1991, p. 467, Table 757.

24. U.S. Senate, "Health Care Access and Affordability Act of 1991," S. 1995, 102d Cong., 1st Sess. (Washington, D.C.: U.S. Government Printing Office, 1991).

Part III

Special Interests, the Law and Political Posturing

8

Special Interests and Legislation

Throughout the 1980s and up to the present time, participation by special interest groups in congressional hearings and special interest group pressures on members of Congress and Cabinet members has been increasing steadily. Scholars, practitioners, business leaders, and even politicians are beginning to complain publicly that special interests have overstepped the bounds of persuasion and have become almost coercive in their dealings with Congress.[1]

It is the privilege, even an obligation, of each citizen to petition Congress, to call to its attention social problems for which Congress can provide a remedy. Increasingly, many proactive special interest groups have taken militant stands regarding a very narrow range of issues that may benefit the few constituents they represent, but may cause millions of other citizens to subsidize their constituents with no direct benefit for themselves in return.[2]

Not all special interest groups take such narrow positions on social issues. As we shall see from the following classification of most special interest groups, some have larger constituencies than others, and therefore take a broader view of social needs than just their own. Almost any categories which are set up will have special exceptions, but they typically may be classified, from those with a broader social focus (providers) to those with very narrow focus (consumers), as:

1. Health Care Providers. This group includes hospitals, physician associations like the AMA, nursing associations, pharmaceutical firms and associations, and other groups closely tied to delivering health care and associated health care goods and services.
2. Payers. This groups includes insurance companies and associations, businesses, state and local governments, and other groups which typically have to pay for health care and associated health care goods and services.
3. Consumer Groups. These groups may typically be subcategorized as:
   (a) associations representing their own members—AARP, NOW, etc.,
   (b) associations and organizations representing categories of society which may not be members at all—aged, poor, blacks, children, disabled, etc., and
   (c) associations and organizations representing specific diseases and conditions—heart disease, cancer, Alzheimer's, AIDS, mental health, etc.

They are all major stakeholders in health care, but they have different objectives and use different tactics to obtain their objectives. Notice that the providers are interested in having individuals and organizations spend more on health care. The consumer special interests are interested in maximizing the amount of health care expenditures for their constituents and also keeping health care costs at the lowest levels throughout the provider network. The payers are interested in keeping all health care costs at a minimum in both the provider and consumer segments of the health care community. It is obvious that the objectives of the various special interests are in conflict with each other. This accounts for the conflicting signals received by Congress on the issue of providing health care to the nation.

A major criticism levelled at the consumer special interest groups is that they are typically non-profit groups, do not produce a product except influence and pressure, hire few, if any, full-time employees, and lobby for very specialized causes. Additionally, whether the leaders of these special interest groups represent the views of their members is a point of controversy among social and political scientists.

LABOR UNIONS AND THE AMA AS LOBBYISTS

What is not common knowledge about the impact of special interests on legislation is the running feud between the American Federation of Labor/Congress of Industrial Organizations (AFL-CIO) labor unions and the American Medical Association (AMA) during the 1950s and 1960s. During this approximate decade, the labor unions were fighting to have the medical costs shifted from the employer to the federal government so that the total wage bill (direct costs of labor plus all benefits, including medical benefits) would not be diminished, leaving more of it for direct worker wages. The strategy was to lobby the government to include Medicare under the Social Security funding. This would shift costs for retiree medical care from the employer to the federal government in the form of Medicare.

The American Medical Association believed that medical care should be tied to income-related programs funded by general tax revenues. Their position was not quite so straightforward as the union's position, since there were two edges to the Medicare sword. If government subsidies were to go only to those who could not afford physician services, the subsidies would create an even greater demand for those services. This was the good part of the program. If, however, the subsidy did not increase the demand much, and if the government subsidy took the place of the private payment, then the program would increase costs to the point that there might be a call for controls to be placed on physician fees. This was not a good part of the program.

To indicate the power of special interests to obtain their goals often at the expense of the general taxpayers, we observe what actually happened with the solution to the tug-of-war between the labor unions and the American Medical Association regarding Medicare:

1. The Social Security vehicle was used as a basis for eligibililty for Medicare, Part B, acceding to pressure from, primarily, the labor unions.[3]
2. The payment system for physicians and hospitals on a ''cost plus'' basis was implemented out of general tax revenues— the burden of which is borne by the total working population. Physicians and hospitals were subsidized by taxpayers—payment guaranteed by the federal and state governments.[4]
3. The working population paid the bill through a) higher taxes

to fund Medicare, Part B, and Medicaid, and b) through higher prices for their own medical services.[5]

Probably the most classic example of the power of special interests to influence legislation is the case of the Medicare Catastrophic Coverage Act of 1988, Public Law 100–360, which was subsequently repealed by the Medicare Catastrophic Coverage Repeal Act, H.R. 3607, in November of 1989.[6] Senator, and later Representative, Claude D. Pepper (D.-FL)—after whom the "Pepper Commission" (U.S. Bipartisan Commission on Comprehensive Health Care) was named—was a champion of health care for the aged,[7] himself being a person in his eighties. He was supported in his efforts to get the Medicare Catastrophic Coverage Act passed by the special interest lobbying efforts of the American Association of Retired Persons (AARP). Once the AARP and other special interests representing the elderly found out that the elderly would have to pay for their benefits, they immediately turned 180 degrees on the issue and began to attack it.

The National Committee to Preserve Social Security and Medicare got its members and the members of the AARP to protest the surtax associated with the Medicare Catastrophic Coverage Act. "The surcharge imposed by Congress was 15 percent on the income taxes of the elderly who had yearly tax liabilities of more than $150 per year. Congress indicated that only about 40 percent of the elders would have paid any tax at all, and only 5 percent would have actually paid the maximum contribution of $800 for individuals or $1,600 for couples."[8] The result of the protest was the repeal of the Medicare Catastrophic Coverage Act, even though some of the provisions of the Act were still preserved in the current Medicare provisions.

Labor unions are, to this day, in a quandary regarding the spiraling cost of health care and the effect that these increasing costs will have on employers. The AFL-CIO ran commercials before the 1992 Democratic and Republican conventions proposing their ideas for better health care coverage. John Sweeney, chairman of the AFL-CIO Health Care Committee and president of the Service Employees International Union (SEIU) presented a checklist of items that he proposed to call to the attention of congressmen and congresswomen before the 1992 elections:

1. Cost shifting among payers occurs when providers charge private plans above cost because public programs pay below cost. The new federal budget includes $32 billion in savings

from reduced payments to providers—every penny of which will show up in increased charges to private plans.

2. Some companies provide no health insurance to their workers. The rest of us pick up the tab through our family coverage plans and through higher charges on our hospital bills.
3. Here's one some of us can control: large plans can negotiate discounts, but the rest of us will pick up the difference.
4. Hospitals and doctors compete with each other by adding new services and installing expensive medical technology. Not much we can do about that.
5. Drug companies use their vast market power to raise prices at will—some 10% a year since 1980.
6. Doctors exercise market power—and quite effectively too. Again, we can have at best only a small impact, and a temporary one at that.
7. And then there's the growing administrative costs, which add to overhead.
8. Finally, there's the waste in the system—evidence that physicians perform large numbers of unnecessary tests and procedures.[9]

Notice that this is just one lobbying effort, but it is composed of over 800,000 members and represents 350 local unions. Being a member of the Benefits Liaison Committee, Sweeney will surely repeat the point made in the article: "Our members have made hundreds of visits to members of Congress to let them know what is happening at the bargaining table. We're also telling Congress that we think the health care cost crisis is the responsibility of the federal government. We aim to make health care reform the number one domestic policy issue in the 1992 Presidential elections."[10]

HEALTH CARE AS A RIGHT

A uniquely explicit statement of health care as a "right" is cited in the Commonwealth of Massachusetts document "An Act to Make Health Security Available to All Citizens of the Commonwealth and to Improve Hospital Financing," which states that access "to basic health care services is a *natural, essential, and unalienable right.*"[11] Buchi and Landesman define two major types of rights, negative rights and positive rights.[12] They argue that negative rights require essentially the *noninterference* on others, while positive rights *require the help and aid* of others to obtain what they have a right to or right to do. Examples of negative rights are the protection of free speech, peaceable enjoyment of property and home, persons and property against police force, and unreasonable intrusion in our lives by the courts. The list could be expanded, but it is sufficient to point out that negative rights are more passive and usually require less in both costs and resources to maintain them.

Positive rights, in contrast, require both programs to provide them and agencies to administer them. Notice that the positive rights require a transfer of wealth from those who have more wealth in life to those who have less. They are, therefore, generally thought to be unpopular and are usually provided with no small amount of resistance from those who have to do the subsidizing. Health care is thought, by some, to be a positive right—one that should have both moral and legal standing and implementation, but this view raises a number of interesting questions, including the following:

1. What is a basic or decent level of health care?
2. Who should have the responsibility to provide health care—physicians, hospitals, institutions, third party payers?
3. Are health care services above a basic level to be distributed as a negative right?
4. Is it a violation of people's property rights to be forced to pay for their own health care and then transfer portions of their wealth to pay for the health care of persons who pay nothing for their health care?[13]

The special interest groups associated with the so-called Pro-Choice and the Pro-Life movements are in literal physical and legal combat over the care associated with abortions. Indigent and poor women typically cannot afford the care associated with an abortion, even though Justice Thurgood Marshall believed that non-emergency medical care was a *basic necessity of life for the poor* and had the same standing as welfare assistance provided to the poor.[14] Generally, however, the justices of the Supreme Court have argued—as in *Maher v. Roe* and *Harris v. McRae*—that state and federal legislatures are not obligated to provide government funds for services for indigent or poor women and that they may deny Medicaid funds for abortion services unless the pregnancy involves a life-threatening situation.[15] Both the Democratic and Republican candidates for President of the United States, in 1992, took strong stands in their respective party platforms regarding the *right* of abortion-related health services.

RIGHTS FOR THE HANDICAPPED AND THE DISABLED

Even before the Americans with Disabilities Act (ADA) of 1990, Public Law 101–336 (Title I, S. 933, 101st Cong. and Title II, H.R. 2773, 101st Cong.),[16] was to become effective in July, 1992, a movement was taking shape to repeal the act. On June 22, 1992, Representative Edwards of Oklahoma introduced and referred H.R. 5450 to the Committees on Education and Labor, Energy and Commerce, Judiciary, and Public Works to repeal the Americans with Disabilities Act of 1990. Since the first debate of the ADA, it became obvious to businesses, industry, and scholars across the spectrum of health and medical care that the ADA, in its enacted form was a major cost shifting maneuver of the Congress to shift the responsibilities and costs of the disabled from Congress to the private sector.

Senate Report No. 116 states that the Americans with Disabilities Act was intended to '' . . . provide a clear and comprehensive national mandate to end discrimination against individuals with disabilities and to bring persons with disabilities into the economic and social mainstream of American life . . . , to provide enforceable standards addressing discrimination against individuals with disabilities, and to ensure that the Federal government plays a central role in enforcing these standards on behalf of individuals with disabilities.''[17]

An individual is considered to be "disabled" if the individual has a physical or mental impairment that substantially limits one or more of the major life activities of the individual, has a history or record of such impairment, or is regarded as having such impairment.

The possibilities for litigation are boundless. For example, being regarded as having a disability refers to an individual who, though not disabled, may be perceived as disabled. What has perplexed businesses and scholars is the inclusion of the infectious disease AIDS in the Americans with Disabilities Act. They argue that if infectious diseases are to be included, then why not include syphilis and gonorrhea, or, perhaps many other non-infectious diseases. The inclusion of AIDS was perceived to be strictly a cost and responsibility shift from the government to the private sector due to extreme AIDS special interest pressure on the members of Congress.[18]

NOTES

1. Thomas Curtis and Donald Westerfield, *Congressional Intent* (New York: Praeger, 1992).

2. Donald Westerfield, *Mandated Health Care: Issues and Strategies* (New York: Praeger, 1991), chapters 2 and 4.

3. U.S. Dept. of Health and Human Services, *The Medicare Handbook* (Baltimore: Health Care Financing Administration, 1989); U.S. House of Representatives, Energy and Commerce Subcommittee on Health and the Environment, *Elder-Care Long-Term Care Assistance Act of 1988*, 100th Cong., 16 September 1988, H.R. 5320; U.S. House of Representatives, Select Committee on Aging, *Building an American Health System: Journey Toward a Healthy and Caring America*, Comm. Pub. No. 101–740, 101st Cong., Jan. 1990; U.S. House of Representatives, Ways and Means Subcommittee on Health, *Chronic Care Medicare Long-Term Care Coverage Act of 1988*, 100th Cong., 27 September 1988, H.R. 5393.

4. Gerard Anderson et al., "Capitation Pricing: Adjusting for Prior Utilization and Physician Discretion," *Health Care Financing Review* (Winter 1986):27–34; also Allen Dobson and Elizabeth Hoy, "Hospital PPS Profits: Past and Prospective," *Health Affairs* (Spring 1988):126–129.

5. Paul Feldstein, *The Politics of Health Legislation: An Economic Perspective* (Ann Arbor, Michigan: Health Administration Press, 1988); see also Marian Gornick et al., "Twenty Years of Medicare and Medicaid: Covered Populations, Use of Benefits, and Program Expenditures," *Health Care Financing Review, 1985 Annual Supplement* (Washington, D.C.: Health Care Financing Association, 1985).

6. Susan Garland, ed., "The Torpedo That Slammed Into Catastrophic Health Care," *Business Week* (23 Oct. 1989):70; see also the wording of U.S. House of Representatives, *Medicare Long-Term Care Catastrophic Protection Act*, 100th Cong., 24 June 1987, H.R. 2762.

7. U.S. Bipartisan Commission on Comprehensive Health Care, *A Call For Action* (Washington, D.C.: U.S. Government Printing Office, 1990).

8. Anetta Miller and Mary Hager, "The Elderly Duke It Out," *Newsweek* (11 Sept. 1989):42–43; see also Donald Westerfield, *Mandated Health Care: Issues and Strategies* (New York: Praeger, 1991), pp. 30–31.

9. John Sweeney, "National Health Care Reform—A Labor Perspective" *Employee Benefits Digest*, International Foundation of Employee Benefit Plans, (February 1991):1, 8.

10. John Sweeney, "National Health Care Reform," *op. cit.*, p. 8.

11. Commonwealth of Massachusetts, "An Act to Make Health Security Available to All Citizens of the Commonwealth and to Improve Hospital Financing," chapter 23 of the acts of 1988.

12. Kenneth Buchi and Bruce Landesman, "Health Care in a National Health Program: A Fundamental Right" in Robert Huefner and Margaret Battin, eds., *Changing to National Health Care: Ethical and Policy Issues* (Salt Lake City, Utah: University of Utah Press, 1992), pp. 191–208; see also the arguments in Allen Buchanan, "Competition, Charity, and the Right to Health Care" in Thomas Attig et al., ed., *The*

Restraint of Liberty (Bowling Green, Ohio: Bowling Green State University, 1985):129–143.

13. James Nickel, *Making Sense of Human Rights* (Berkeley, California: University of California Press, 1987).

14. *Memorial Hospital v. Maricopa County*, 415 U.S. 250 (1974).

15. See the text of *Maher v. Roe*, 432 U.S. 464 (1977) *Harris v. McRae*, 448 U.S. 297 (1980); and the so-called "Hyde Amendment," Public Law 96–123, sec. 109.

16. Americans with Disabilities Act of 1990, Public Law 101–336 (Title I, S. 933, 101st Cong. and Title II, H.R. 2773, 101st Cong.).

17. U.S. Senate, Senate Report No. 116, 101st Cong., 1st. Sess. (1989). Refer also to the Senate version of the Americans with Disabilities Act, S. 933, 101st Cong., sec. 102(a) (1989).

18. Jane West, "Introduction—Implementing the Act: Where We Begin," *The Milbank Quarterly* Supp. 1/2, 69 (1991):xi–xxxi; See also Jane West, "The Social and Policy Context of the Act," *The Milbank Quarterly* Supp. 1/2, 69 (1991):3–24; Richard J. Donahue, "AIDS Cost Could Lead to National Health Insurance Plan," *National Underwriter* (9 Nov. 1987):6, 46; Brian Harrigan and Nancy Jones, "The Cost Impact of AIDS on Employee Benefits Programs," *Compensation & Benefits Management* Vol. 3 (Winter 1987):27–29.

9

The Law—Federal Mandates

It is impossible to understand the direction that proposed health care legislation should take until the course of past federal mandates has been studied. From the previous chapter, one is able to see how pressures from literally hundreds of special interest groups are translated into federal mandates that often benefit only a select target group. It is clear that special interests, lobbyists, and political action committees influence, and often distort, the perception of public need in the eyes of legislators. The result has been that congressional priorities do not match the priorities and needs of those who ultimately bear the greatest burden of the federal mandates. This is especially true in health care, where the ones who need help most have the least voice in and access to congressional committees.

The old saying: "The squeaky wheel gets the oil" is true, but does it quit squeaking even after getting some oil? Does it require even greater doses once it has successfully squeaked loudly and obtained oil in the first place? Experience with pressure groups has proven that with each success in lobbying Congress, these groups apply even greater pressure to obtain further consideration and concessions to their causes. Is this in the public interest? These are difficult questions because someone actually does benefit from these lobbying efforts. The question to be answered, however, is whether the benefits to a few are worth the costs to the others who benefit little or not at all.

The laws discussed in this chapter are those which have directly or indirectly grown out of the so-called "great society" programs during and shortly after the administration of President Lyndon Johnson. Some of the laws appear, on the surface, not to be directly related to health care, but they have laid the foundation for precedents and legislation which are contained in the main body of current health care legislation and proposals.

THE CIVIL RIGHTS ACT

The Department of Health and Human Services (DHHS) provides health care services to hospitals, primary care facilities, outpatient clinics, state and local public health agencies, day care centers, and countless local service agencies and programs. They all receive federal funds for the provision of those services. Title VI, Section 601, of the Civil Rights Act of 1964 states, in part: "No persons in the United States shall, on the grounds of race, color, or national origin, be excluded from participation, or be denied benefits of, or be subjected to racial discrimination under any program or activity receiving Federal financial assistance."[1]

After the enactment of the Civil Rights Act, Medicare and Medicaid, Titles XVII and XIX of the Social Security Act of 1965, the Department of Health, Education and Welfare (HEW), which became the Department of Health and Human Services (DHHS) began to increase its enforcement activities under Title VI.[2] It should be remembered that the Office of Civil Rights (OCR) was under the Department of Health and Human Services and was charged with enforcing the statutory enforcement of Title VI and its programs.

A complaint under the Title VI provisions is filed according to the procedure outlined below:

Under Title VI a complainant must make an oral or written allegation to OCR within 180 days of the last act of alleged discrimination 'unless the time limitation is waived for good cause by the designated OCR official.' Oral allegations must be reduced to writing. The filing day limitation is not applicable to complainants who allege continuing violations or to Hill-Burton community service complainants. OCR regional offices have 195 calendar days from the date of receipt of a complete complaint to make a compliance determination or, when necessary, to forward to OCR Headquarters on enforcement recommendation.[3]

It is interesting to note that there were almost no health care complaints processed by the Office of Civil Rights during the early 1970s due to the heavy litigation in the education field. Complaints regarding discrimination in educational facilities, busing children to other schools, assignment of children to schools according to quotas, and alleged discrimination in discipline and grading occupied most of the resources of the OCR until the mid- to late-1970s.

HILL-BURTON HOSPITAL SURVEY AND CONSTRUCTION ACT

It seems very unlikely that the Hill-Burton Hospital Survey and Construction Act of 1946[4] would have even the remotest relationship to the enforcement of civil rights complaints in health care. This act was originally passed to provide funds to build hospitals, to provide for formal planning of health care facilities, and for the maintenance of quality in health care facilities. It was used primarily to set standards for state hospital licensing laws as well as the standards for health care facilities.[5]

When a civil rights complaint involves alleged discrimination in community services, the Office of Civil Rights usually seeks to obtain voluntary compliance. If it is not successful in obtaining the voluntary compliance, the director of the Office of Civil Rights must refer the complaint directly to the U.S. Department of Justice for further action. Even though the relative number of complaints filed under the Hill-Burton regulations is small, they, nevertheless, have been instrumental in laying the foundation for legal precedents and administrative opinions that are reflected in current health care mandates which have jurisdictions throughout the hospital facilities network in the United States.

The Hill-Burton story is a mixed story. It helped shape the authority for the federal government to extend its interests into hospitals and community services, but its reputation was somewhat tarnished by being associated with congressional ''pork barrel'' projects. Kenneth Wing describes both the success and shortcomings of the Hill-Burton agencies:

It has been estimated that in the first 20 years of the program more than half of the hospitals in the country received Hill-Burton assistance . . . Yet its success highlights its shortcomings. . . . Hill-Burton agencies could only encourage necessary modernization and construction. They had no authority to curb unnecessary projects. . . . Hill-Burton, particularly in its later years, has been described by some critics as a 'pork barrel' program, contributing as much to the oversupply of hospital beds as to the rationalization or planned distribution of necessary health facilities.[6]

AGE DISCRIMINATION IN EMPLOYMENT ACT

The Age Discrimination in Employment Act (ADEA) of 1967, was later amended by both the Tax Equity and Fiscal Responsibility Act (TEFRA) of 1982 and the Deficit Reduction Act (DEFRA) of 1984.[7] This act prohibits discrimination with respect to age for individuals between the ages of 40 years and 70 years. The purpose of the legislation was to give persons who are perceived to be "older" a chance to come into or remain in the labor force based on their ability, without regard to age. It was a well-meaning piece of legislation, but it was not well thought out. It has tried to solve one of the social problems of aging by mandating that employers hire or retain workers, usually 60 or above in practice, without regard to their potential for productivity.

By requiring employers to retain employees who would normally be retiring at or about 60 years of age, the employer is forced to retain those employees whose health care costs are typically at a maximum. While many of those persons past 60 years of age are still productive, there are industries in which persons at or above 60 years cannot be productive without the employer's making excessive accommodations to the older employees which are unfair to less senior employees who are usually making much less in salary or wages.

This law, while passed with the best of social intentions, shifts at least the following costs to the employer:

1. Increased costs of health care and benefits.
2. Salary differentials between older employees' salaries and younger employees' salaries for the same job or level of productivity.
3. Decreased productivity through discrimination as perceived through the eyes of younger employees who may be more productive and make lower wages.
4. Increased absenteeism due to health problems.

The Age Discrimination in Employment Act led to TEFRA and DEFRA, as mentioned above. Those two acts, discussed in more detail below, mandated that employers provide the same health care benefits to employees and their spouses, aged 65 to 70, that are provided to younger employees, irrespective of costs or utilization. Additionally, *Medicare was mandated to be the secondary payer* to the employer's health care benefits package, that is, the employer's health care plan must pay the first dollars of health care even though those identical benefits would be paid through Medicare.

REHABILITATION ACT

It is interesting to follow the thread of various federal mandates to the present time, especially when the earlier mandates seem, on the surface, to be only tangentially related to the issue at hand. The Rehabilitation Act of 1973, however, provided the foundation to one of the most controversial bills to be passed by Congress—the Americans With Disabilities Act.[8] This act broadened the scope of federal jurisdiction to virtually every person doing business with the federal government or receiving contracts valued at least at $2,500. Jane West describes certain sections of the act as follows:

In 1973, sections 501, 503, and 504 were enacted as part of the Rehabilitation Act. Section 504 prohibits discrimination against otherwise qualified persons with disabilities in any program activity receiving federal funds and in executive agencies and the Postal Service. Sections 501 and 503 require affirmative-action plans for the hiring and advancement of persons with disabilities in the federal government and any contractors receiving federal contracts over $2,500. Section 504 is the most significant building block for the ADA [Americans with Disabilities Act]. Its 17-year history of implementation has delineated many core concepts of the ADA, such as 'reasonable accommodation' and 'undue burden.' Numerous court decisions have examined questions raised by section 504, such as how to determine when a person with a disability is 'otherwise qualified,' when a 'reasonable accommodation' crosses the line and becomes an 'undue burden,' and when a person with a disability presents a threat to the health and/or safety of others.[9]

It is impossible to obtain a solid number of workers covered by the Rehabilitation Act and the subsequent Americans with Disabilities Act, but the two concepts from the Rehabilitation Act that had the greatest impact on business were the concepts of ''otherwise qualified'' and ''reasonable accommodation.'' These concepts opened the door for the government to mandate that the burden of proof is on the employer when a person with a disability is not accepted for employment or is displaced from a current position or one which the disabled person desires. Yelin assesses the impact of Section 504 of the Rehabilitation Act thusly: ''Because section 504 served as a model for the Americans with Disabilities Act, its impact on employment in the intervening years may prove a bellwether for the ADA.''[10]

TEFRA AND DEFRA

Even though the legislation discussed up to this point may be controversial with regard to impact and who should bear the ultimate burden, one could rationalize their enactment by acknowledging that health care coverage was extended to a greater number of persons. That does not resolve the question regarding whether health care is the responsibility of the various levels of government or the responsibility of employers. The Siamese twins of TEFRA, the Tax Equity and Fiscal Responsibility Act of 1982, and DEFRA, the Deficit Reduction Act of 1984, flagrantly shifted the costs of health care which would normally be covered by Medicare, for those workers aged 65 through 69, from the federal government to the employer.[11]

The Tax Equity and Fiscal Responsibility Act amended the Age Discrimination in Employment Act of 1967 to require employers to offer employees age 65 through 69 the same coverage under the same plans as was offered to employees under age 65. As Westerfield argued:

TEFRA shifted a significant portion of the social welfare costs of the 65 through 69 age group to the employer by requiring the employer to provide group health coverage to that age group despite the considerations that:

1. They would otherwise be covered under Medicare.
2. Their medical costs were many times higher than the lower age groups.
3. Most of the persons in that age group probably could not qualify for group coverage otherwise due to their health profile.

   4. It contradicted sound underwriting principles.
   5. It had immediate negative influence on business earnings.[12]

Two years later, Congress mandated the Deficit Reduction Act of 1984 (DEFRA). This mandate required employers to provide the same benefits under the same plans for *spouses* aged 65 through 69 of the employees covered under TEFRA. The same arguments outlined in the preceding paragraph are also valid for the spouses. What is even more flagrant about this cost shifting from the federal government to the employer is that the spouses of the employees aged 65 through 69 do not participate in any productive activity for the employer.[13]

By mandating that those employees and their spouses aged 65 through 69 have Medicare as secondary payer, the government indicated to business and industry that it could and would shift its social and financial responsibilities to employers irrespective of the costs. Recall that there was no provision for added compensation to the employers for the added premium and administrative costs of this mandated liability. It is this action and the Age Discrimination in Employment Act (ADEA) that has caused business and industry to resist further federal mandates in health care. Additionally, employers find that the added costs are requiring adjustments in their workforce, requiring the elimination of marginal jobs. These marginal jobs are held by persons who need health care benefits the most.

AMERICANS WITH DISABILITIES ACT

Perhaps the most controversial bill passed by Congress in recent times, the Americans with Disabilities Act (ADA) of 1990 has caused a bonanza for lawyers and litigation.[14] The act was designed with good intentions:

   1. Disabled persons should have equal access to jobs if they are "otherwise qualified" for them.
   2. If the disability prevents a disabled person from performing the duties of the job, "reasonable accommodations" must be made in order to enable the disabled person to do so.

To the disabled person, this act was a blessing, literally. To business and industry, the act created a hellish legal nightmare and placed the government between the employer and applicants for jobs and between the supervisor responsible for productivity and scheduling and the employee. The definition of a disability is itself grounds for endless litigation. The Americans with Disabilities Act defines a disabled person as someone who:

1. Has a physical or mental impairment that substantially limits that person in one or more major life activities, or
2. Has a record of such a physical or mental impairment, or
3. Is regarded as having such a physical or mental impairment.

As we view the Americans with Disabilities Act, it would be good to keep in mind that there are at least two views of the issue—*who must pay and who benefits*. Title I of the ADA requires that employers make "reasonable accommodations" to the persons with disabilities (either already qualified or as a means of enabling them to be qualified) unless the employer "can demonstrate that the accommodation will impose an *undue hardship* in terms of difficulty or expense." Notice that the employer must prove that the disabled person cannot do the job without reasonable accommodation. This means that the employer must provide the accommodation at least in terms of:

1. Specialized equipment.
2. Altered environment.
3. Adjustments in work schedule.
4. Sequence of events required to do the job.
5. Different combinations of people, equipment, and procedures.

Rate of pay and health care benefits are supposed to be the same for the disabled person for whom accommodations are made and the non-disabled person. The costs per man hour of work will be greater for the disabled person. Even after the employer makes "good faith" attempts to "accommodate" the disabled person, it may be found that the job cannot be reconfigured within reasonable costs. Thomas Chirikos discusses the economics of employing persons with disabilities and finds that:

. . . persons with disabilities who enter the labor force post ADA are likely to be more severely impaired than those currently employed, therefore requiring more expensive accommodation. When people with disabilities are working, it clearly benefits the economy; however, the cost to individual businesses may be prohibitive in certain circumstances.[15]

Persons with AIDS are included within the definition of persons with disabilities. This means that they must be given accommodation considerations in both job application and on the job. Can it be reasonable to expect a full career from a person who has been diagnosed as having AIDS? The life expectancy is less than three years, yet the employer must hire that person if that person is otherwise qualified. Can the health care costs associated with a person with AIDS be comparable to a person without AIDS? No, the costs are many times higher. Is there a risk of transmitting AIDS to other persons on the job? The risks of transmission are unknown, but it is known that risk is not zero.

This act was mandated on employers as part of a national plan to provide employment and health care to those with disabilities. While it would be unusual to find a person who would disagree with the underlying notion that these persons can be productive and can make a positive contribution to the economy, it would also be unusual to find a person who would agree that the employer should bear the burden of these social welfare costs. The federal, state, and local governments have responsibilities for the social welfare of taxpayers and other citizens. The employers do not have such a responsibility. This social welfare "cost shifting" has prompted efforts in the U.S. House of Representatives to repeal this act. Whether the social benefits equal the social costs of this act is yet to be determined.

H.R. 5450—REPEAL THE ADA

In discussing the Americans with Disabilities Act, it is important to remember that, like all legislation passed by Congress, it too has its opponents. H.R. 5450 To Repeal the Americans with Disabilities Act is presented on the following page to indicate the nature of a bill to repeal another bill and to exhibit a bill from the U.S. House of Representatives. Notice that the actual language for repeal is only ten words.

Figure 9.1
H.R. 5450

102D CONGRESS
2D SESSION
H. R. 5450

To repeal the Americans with Disabilities Act of 1990.

IN THE HOUSE OF REPRESENTATIVES

JUNE 22, 1992

Mr. EDWARDS of Oklahoma introduced the following bill; which was referred jointly to the Committees on Education and Labor, Energy and Commerce, Public Works and Transportation, and the Judiciary

A BILL

To repeal the Americans with Disabilities Act of 1990.

1   *Be it enacted by the Senate and House of Representa-*

2 *tives of the United States of America in Congress assembled,*

3 That the Americans with Disabilities Act of 1990 (Public

4 Law   –336; 42 U.S.C. 12101 et seq.) is repealed.

O

NOTES

1. Civil Rights Act of 1964, P.L. 88–352, Title VI, Section 601. This Act was amended by the bill introduced by Representative Brooks to the U.S. House of Representatives on January 3, 1991, as the "Civil Rights and Women's Equity in Employment Act of 1991," H.R. 1, 102d Cong., 1st Sess.; see also Westerfield's discussion of the maneuvering for this bill in Thomas Curtis and Donald Westerfield, *Congressional Intent* (New York: Praeger, 1992), pp. 52–53.

2. Woodrow Jones and Mitchell Rice, eds., *Health Care Issues in Black America: Policies, Problems, and Prospects* (New York: Greenwood Press, 1987), pp. 100–101; See also U.S. House of Representatives, H.R. Doc. No. 318, 88th Cong., 2nd Sess. (Washington, D.C.: U.S. Government Printing Office, 1964).

3. Jones and Rice, *Health Care Issues in Black America, op. cit.*, p. 102.

4. See P.L. 79–725, 60 Stat. 1040 (1970); 42 U.S.C. subjects. 291(a)–291(p).

5. Ruth Roemer and George McKay, *Legal Aspects of Health Policy: Issues and Trends* (Westport, Connecticut: Greenwood Press, 1980), pp. 37–38.

6. Kenneth Wing, *The Law and the Public's Health* 3rd ed. (Ann Arbor, Michigan: Health Administration Press, 1990), pp. 147–148.

7. George Pozgar, *Legal Aspects of Health Care Administration* 4th ed. (Rockville, Maryland: Aspen Publishers, 1990), p. 220; and *1991 Guidebook to Fair Employment Practices* Sec. 112.6 "Age Discrimination" (Chicago: Commerce Clearing House, 1991), pp. 22–23. See also a discussion of TEFRA and DEFRA in Donald Westerfield, *Mandated Health Care: Issues and Strategies* (New York: Praeger, 1991), pp. 26–27 and Rory Albert and Neal Schelberg, "Benefit Plans Redefined Under ADEA; Cases and Rulings," *Pension World* (October 1989):45–48.

8. Rehabilitation Act of 1973, 29 U.S.C. chapter 14 and the Americans With Disabilities Act P.L. 101–336, 104 Stat. 327, 42 U.S.C. 12101 sec.2.; see also Jane West, ed., *The Americans with Disabilities Act: From Policy to Practice* (New York: Milbank Memorial Fund, 1991).

9. Jane West, ed., "The Social and Policy Context of the Act" in *The Americans with Disabilities Act: From Policy to Practice, op. cit.*, pp. 16–17; see also 29 U.S.C. 791–794.

10. Edward Yelin, "The Recent History and Immediate Future of Employment among Persons with Disabilities" in Jane West, ed., *The Americans with Disabilities Act: From Policy to Practice, op. cit.*, p. 136; see also *1991 Guidebook to Fair Employment Practices* Sec. 112.7, "Handicap Discrimination Under Rehabilitation Act" (Chicago: Commerce Clearing House, 1991), pp. 23–24.

11. Donald Westerfield, *Mandated Health Care: Issues and Strategies* (New York: Praeger, 1991); Donald Westerfield and Paul Wilson, "Employers and the Medicare Secondary Payer: IRS/SSA/HCFA Data Match Project," *Proceedings of the Business and Health Administration Association* (March 1992):127–130.

12. Donald Westerfield, *Mandated Health Care, op. cit.*, pp. 26–27.

13. Paul Wilson and Donald Westerfield, "Is Shifting Health Care Costs the Right Strategy for the U.S.?" *NAEDA Journal* (December 1990):9–12; Jack Bresch and Frederick Krebs, "Compulsory Employee Benefits: Pro And Con," *Association Management* (April 1989):86–91; L. Dosier and L. Hamilton, "Social Responsibility and Your Employer," *Personnel Administrator* (Apr. 1989):88, 90, 92, 95.

14. Americans with Disabilities Act of 1990, Public Law 101–336 (Title I, S. 933, 101st Cong. and Title II, H.R. 2773, 101st Cong.).

15. Thomas Chirikos, ''The Economics of Employment'' in Jane West, ed., *The Americans with Disabilities Act: From Policy to Practice* (New York: Milbank Memorial Fund, 1991):150.

10

Obstacles Faced By Small Businesses

The imprint of the special interests on health care legislation throughout the 1980s and into the 1990s is indelible. The maneuvering and posturing of the hundreds of special interest groups and their lobbyists have created chaos in the legislative committees of Congress.[1] The legislation that actually became the law, as discussed in the previous chapter, reflects a cut-and-paste hodgepodge of amendments designed more to placate powerful special interests and help ensure re-election than a carefully designed strategy to provide the best health care possible to the widest range of citizens at the lowest possible cost. This has resulted in undue burdens on small businesses, gaps in health care coverage for elders and the underprivileged, and spiraling health care costs.[2]

Political debate on the floors of the U.S. Senate and the U.S. House of Representatives reflect the difficulty in obtaining a consensus measure from the fragmented congressional committees. This is magnified by the activities of the professional staff contingents of each of the congressmen and congresswomen, who have professional backgrounds and aspirations which are often at variance with the member of Congress for whom they work.[3] Even to the constituencies for whom a legislative measure was designed, the resulting public law seems to be like the description of the old-fashioned hoop skirt—"covers all, touches nothing."

Of over thirty legislative health care proposals discussed in chapters 5 through 7 of this book, it is unlikely that any of them will be passed in a form acceptable to the health care providers, insurers, health care administrators, or especially those who are desperate for health care insurance coverage of any kind. In testimony before the Committee on Education and Labor in the U.S. House of Representatives, Representative Richard Armey (R.-TX) stated:

> There isn't a problem in the world that isn't so bad that we can't make it worse. Undoubtedly the explosion in health care costs is the most critical issue facing business and labor. The rate of increase is truly unsustainable. But if we pursue the wrong reform plan, we will do nothing to provide affordable health care to all of our people. We will instead author an economic disaster.[4]

COST SHIFTING TO PRIVATE SECTOR

The quotation from Representative Armey is prophetic. Because legislation in the last fifteen years has been so completely dominated by the influence of special interests, a legislative consensus is almost impossible to reach. One method that Congress has found to obtain passage of legislation in the health care area is to incrementally mandate health care benefits on employers. In some cases, tax relief is used as a "sweetener" to coax business into minimizing its resistance to the mandates.[5] Despite this relief, the tax consideration is never equal to the added cost of the mandate, therefore the effect of the mandate is to drive costs higher than they were before the mandate was imposed by the government.

In passing the health care mandates, Congress argues that the measures will provide benefits to a larger constituency or will provide more benefits to an already existing constituency. As it actually turns out, the target recipient of the mandated benefits may be worse off than before the mandates for several reasons:

1. Marginal employees, who need the benefits most, are usually the most vulnerable to layoff when it is determined that the total wage bill is excessive.[6]
2. Mandated benefits arbitrarily replace dollar compensation in the total compensation package. Workers with low wages may prefer the dollars to the mandated benefits.[7]
3. Mandated benefits usually do not match the needs of most of the workers, that is, the mandates come from Congress in a "one size fits all" package, without regard to the particular needs of the firm or a specialized industry.
4. Mandated benefits create legal discrimination in the sense that

some employees will never benefit from the mandate. For example, men and women who cannot bear children will not receive maternity benefits, but they must share the costs of such benefits with those who receive them. Similarly, child care benefits to singles and couples without children would not help them.[8]

5. Mandating specific benefits precludes an employee from obtaining the best bundle of benefits and dollars that would otherwise be obtainable from the employer. Needs of employees change with their current lifestyle and economic profile.[9]

The list could be multiplied many times over, but it is sufficient to suggest here that federal mandates are sufficiently inflexible and that individual needs are substituted for the needs of the targeted group. Additionally, there is no guarantee that the group consensus need will bear a close relationship to the specific needs of any given individual within the target group.

In the "Health Care Briefing Paper" prepared by the Joint Economic Committee, the committee argues:

The important point is that in the absence of mandated wages and benefits, employees and employers will tend to arrive at total compensation bundles that are mutually beneficial for both parties to the exchange. Legislating the terms of exchange, either via minimum wage rates or mandatory health plan coverage, restricts individual ability to choose or negotiate the optimum combination of wages and benefits. Employers are told that new health insurance is currency that must be used to pay workers. Workers are told by government that when they sell their labor services, they must accept health insurance as partial payment.

For the employee, the value of the compensation bundle foregone will be greater than the new bundle containing the mandated benefit. If this were not the case, then workers and employers would have agreed on providing the benefit without the mandate. Since benefits are mandated, we can only conclude that they are worth less to the worker than the benefits replaced by government interference in the exchange process. Low-wage, less-skilled workers will bear a disproportionate burden from the new mandate, thus, those workers who the legislation seeks to help are the very workers who are most hurt. The newly imposed health care mandate increases the cost of hiring the targeted worker.[10]

As has been suggested already in the chapter on play or pay, shifting the costs of the mandates associated with play-or-pay will result in a possible 712,742 jobs lost in the economy, but the very small firms, those with less than 20 employees, would account for losses of 308,265 of those jobs.[11] These are firms most likely to hire the lower-waged workers, yet these are the firms which are most vulnerable to the effects of the cost shifting associated with the mandates. The "mandated tax" would be imposed per worker, irrespective of the number of hours worked by that worker or the worker's hourly labor cost.

In a time when global competition for American products overseas is becoming more crucial to our economy, the effect of increased labor costs on potential export products can be chilling. Increased labor costs, especially in the less skilled labor group, means that there are more options for the substitution of capital for labor, especially robotics and automated machinery. As labor is displaced by capital, it is unlikely that the less skilled workers will immediately qualify for other jobs. Their marketable skills have fewer market alternatives, yet they are the most vulnerable to any displacement due to cost shifting from the federal government to the employer.

In testimony before the U.S. House of Representatives Committee on Education and Labor, "Oversight Hearing on National Health Care Reform," Daniel Heslin, Corporate Director of Employee Benefit Programs for Rockwell International Corporation, stated:

Most of the bills introduced so far during the 102nd Congress represent *financing* reform, not *system* reform. Their primary goal is to shift responsibility for payment through government regulation of financing, insurance rating and underwriting, and related issues. They pay scant attention to the way health care itself is organized and delivered.

These bills offer most Americans little or no improvement over their current coverage. No wonder they balk at the notion of paying higher taxes to finance expansion of coverage. ERIC agrees that imposing expanded financing and universal access on top of the deficiencies of the current system's infrastructure will cause a loss of quality, efficiency and cost-effectiveness in the long term.[12]

VULNERABILITY OF SMALL BUSINESS

Most of the health care-related legislation coming out of Congress has been influenced primarily by special interest groups for their respective narrow constituencies. One source of pressure on Congress that is a bit more subtle, yet just as influential in shaping legislation, is the "large business" or so-called "Fortune 500" lobby. The influence of big business is more transparent because big business does not generally like to draw attention to itself, especially when it stands to gain while others lose from a given legislative measure.[13]

When health care legislation is scheduled for debate in the U.S. House of Representatives or in the U.S. Senate, the large firms with a full-time lobbying staff will be aware of the time and place of each meeting. That staff will also have a list of probable witnesses for and against a given issue. The small businesses would not even be able to afford the airfare and all associated expenses of attending such a hearing, would not be able to afford to take the time off from the business for such a hearing, and would probably not know about it in the first place. Additionally, the small firm would not have the resources to produce testimony with the kind of research and documentation necessary to have any influence on the committee.

What this really means is that the normal way for the small business to learn of developments in Congress that will affect their business is through the news media and from an occasional trade paper article. They can only hope that their views will somehow be carried to Congress by the large businesses and by organizations like the National Federation of Independent Business. When John Motley, of that Federation, testified before the Long-Term Strategies For Health Care hearings before the Committee on Ways and Means of the U.S. House of Representatives, he spread before the Committee some major sources of vulnerability with regard to health care costs:

> Two thirds of small businesses offer health insurance. In general, these firms tend to be more mature, more profitable, and have more full-time employees than their counterparts that do not offer health insurance. Despite being fairly stable, these small firms experience high initial premiums and highest renewal premiums. Frequently-cited reasons for the high cost of health insurance for small firms include:
>
> • Insurer fear of adverse selection
> • Instability of the firm

- Lack of expert help in choosing plans
- Little negotiating clout
- Strict experience rating
- Nature of the small business work force
  - labor intensive
  - high percentage of part-time employees
  - high percentage of older workers
  - high percentage of very young workers
  - more remedial workers
  - high turnover
- High administrative costs for the carrier
- Insufficient experience data
- Absence of preferential treatment afforded to larger firms
- Imposition of state premium taxes and mandates[14]

This is a formidable list of obstacles for the small firm to overcome in trying to provide and continue providing health care benefits to its employees. Notice that most of these areas of vulnerability are out of the control of the small business. These forces are exogenous, for the most part, and create an unfavorable rate climate for the small firm. The firm's vulnerability is magnified as the size of the firm becomes smaller. Cost containment measures have to be modest at best. Due to the small firm's size, it is not able to obtain the benefits of self-insuring.

Due to the makeup of the labor market faced by the small firm, workers come into the firm and go out of the firm on an irregular basis, creating a "churning" effect on any insurance plan that the employer may have. Managed care as a cost containment measure is all but impossible, due to the lack of experienced persons to implement such measures. Just the tracking of COBRA beneficiaries places a burden on the small firm that makes its COBRA costs many times the 2 percent margin allowed for administration of the COBRA coverage.

Compliance with both state and federal health care mandates is an administrative nightmare for the small firm. Usually the manager or owner will have a small desk area set aside from the business area where much of the compliance responsibilities are shared with temporary employees or with an employee whose primary work responsibilities are not administrative. For example, in a small clothes shop, it is not unusual to find the manager's desk in a small room not much larger than a closet with absolute minimal office furnishings and supplies. The manager or owner will have business papers mixed together on a "first-come, first-served" basis; hardly an environment in which to battle with complex federal and state health care reform measures.

In the John Motley testimony, cited above, he presents a list of reasons why small firms that do not offer health insurance are not able to do so. The list is probably one of the most persuasive arguments for not implementing the health care reforms proposed in Congress that are based on the employer's offering a government-designed health care package or pay the federal government for not offering one. The items listed by Motley are:

- Cost of premiums or past increases too great
- Insufficient profits
- Insufficient cash flow
- Employee turnover too great
- Too many employees covered elsewhere—secondary wage earners
- Too many part-time employees
- Too many older employees
- Employees prefer cash compensation
- Too small to receive group "discounts"
- No suitable cost-containment options available

This is a list designed by grass-roots analysts and represents realistic impediments to offering and maintaining a health care plan. It serves to dramatize the plight of small businesses in being entrapped in what might be thought of as an endless cycle of "negative returns to smallness."

COBRA AND ERISA

Title I of the Employee Retirement Income Security Act of 1974 (ERISA) was designed to set minimum standards for pension plans in business and industry.[16] It was amended in 1984 by the Retirement Equity Act (REA) and in 1986 by the Tax Reform Act (TRA). ERISA covers:

1. Age and service requirements for eligibility for pension plan participation.
2. For workers with specified minimum employment, vesting benefit accrual, and break in service provisions.
3. Funding provisions—Provisions linked in with COBRA which have the most direct impact on the financial condition of businesses.

4. Fiduciary provisions.
5. Reporting and disclosure provisions.
6. Protection of spouses of pensioners through joint and survivor provisions.

Title X (P.L. 99–272) of the Consolidated Omnibus Budget Reconciliation Act of 1986 (COBRA) amended Title I of ERISA (a new Part 6 was added) to require that group health plans of covered employers provide employees and certain of their family members and dependents with the opportunity to continue health care coverage where coverage under the group health plan would otherwise be terminated.[17] Parallel changes were made in the Internal Revenue Code of 1954 (IRC) and the Public Health Service Act (PHSA).

The spouse and dependent children of covered employees may elect COBRA "continuation coverage" if coverage under an approved plan was last due to:

1. Death of spouse or parent.
2. Termination of spouse's or parent's employment (for reasons other than gross misconduct) or reduction in the spouse's or parent's hours of employment.
3. Divorce or legal separation of spouse or parent.
4. Parent or spouse becomes eligible for Medicare.
5. The dependent ceases to be a "dependent child" under the employer health plan.

Title X of COBRA amended the Internal Revenue Code, Section 162(i), to deny business expense deductions for contributions to any group health plan maintained by the employer unless all the group health plans of the employer meet the continuation coverage requirements of the new IRC Section 162(k).

A new title was added to the Public Health Service Act, Title XXII, which requires that, if a state receives PHSA funds, each group health plan maintained by that state, any political subdivision of that state, or any agency or instrumentality of that state or political subdivision, must provide COBRA continuation coverage under the threat of legal action. The administrative allowance from the federal government for administering the COBRA coverage is 2 percent of the COBRA premium, that is, the total COBRA premium is the base premium plus 2 percent administration fee. The National Federation of Independent Business (NFIB) argues, before the U.S. House of Representatives Ways and Means Committee, that the 2 percent administration fee is far from adequate to cover COBRA administrative costs for small businesses. The NFIB testifies that:

> Studies indicate that the COBRA beneficiary greatly exceed the cost of the premium plus 2 percent. In fact, the average cost is in the neighborhood of an additional 51 percent with many beneficiaries costing the former employer a great deal more. Not only is the business subsidizing the COBRA beneficiaries' additional costs, so are the *current* employees, who many times share in the expense of premium increases. The COBRA Reform Coalition has even documented one situation where over 10 current employees and their families lost coverage because of the cost of one COBRA beneficiary.

It is not unusual for a former employer to receive a COBRA premium paid by a current employer for one of its new employees. What this means is that the former employer may have to provide "continuation" coverage for a separated employee for up to 18 months even though that separated employee is now working for another employer. It is a ludicrous loophole that was designed into COBRA through its "one size fits all" approach. This is only one example of legislation that has been an almost insurmountable obstacle to obtaining a health care policy consensus from business and industry leaders.

Any national plan implemented through employer participation will have to have a strategy that recognizes the special problems faced by small business. The very large firms have enough flexibility in finances, human resources, and power to absorb many of the mandates imposed on business by all levels of government. There are definitely decreasing returns to smallness. Limitations on all resources, small operating margins, inability to stay informed regarding legislative proposals, and limited or no participation in the legislative process in Congress place small business at risk. As we turn, in the next part of this book, to a consideration of an overall national health care strategy, the impact on small businesses must be held paramount, especially if they will share in the heavy burden imposed on them by federal mandates and reforms.

NOTES

1. Thomas Curtis and Donald Westerfield, *Congressional Intent* (New York: Praeger, 1992); Elizabeth Graddy, "Interest Groups or the Public Interest—Why Do We Regulate

Health Occupations?'' *Journal of Health Politics, Policy and Law* (Spring 1991):25–49; Susan Garland, ed., ''The Torpedo That Slammed Into Catastrophic Health Care,'' *Business Week* (23 Oct. 1989):70.

2. Stuart Butler, ''Using Tax Credits to Create an Affordable National Health System,'' *The Heritage Foundation Backgrounder* No. 777 (20 July 1990); Kevin Anderson, ''Small Firms are Getting Squeezed Out,'' *USA Today*, 13 June 1991, pp.1B-2B; ''The Crisis in Health Insurance,'' *Consumer Reports* (Aug. 1990):533–549.

3. See Curtis and Westerfield, *Congressional Intent, op. cit.*, especially chapter 5; Edwin Feulner, Jr., *The Story of the Republican Study Committee: Conservatives Stalk the Congress, 1970–1982* (Ottowa, Ill.: Green Hill Publishers, 1983).

4. Representative Richard Armey (R.-TX) remarks before U.S. House of Representatives, *Oversight Hearing on National Health Care Reform*, Serial No. 102–104, 7 May 1992 (Washington, D.C.: U.S. Government Printing Office, 1992), p. 2.

5. Stuart Butler, ''Using Tax Credits to Create an Affordable National Health System,'' *The Heritage Foundation Backgrounder* No. 777 (20 July 1990); Stuart Butler and Edmund Haislmaier, *A National Health System for America* (Washington, D.C.: The Heritage Foundation, 1989).

6. ''Employers Would Cut Wages, Benefits, If Minimum Health Care Bill Becomes Law,'' *Benefits Today* (6 Nov. 1987):384; Woodrow Jones and Mitchell Rice, eds., *Health Care Issues in Black America: Policies, Problems, and Prospects* (New York: Greenwood Press, 1987); Judy K. Krueger, ''Mandated Health Care And Small Business: Does Anyone Win?'' *Mid America Insurance* (July 1988):26–30.

7. Joel Cantor, ''Expanding Health Insurance Coverage: Who Will Pay?'' *Journal of Health Politics, Policy and Law* (Winter 1990):755–778.

8. Joan Clay, ''The Child Care Issue: Benefits Required By A Changing Workforce,'' *Employee Benefits Journal* (Sept. 1989):32–34; ''Congress Considers Family Leaves,'' *Business Insurance* (2 Apr. 1990):6.

9. R. D. Heller, ''Cafeteria Benefits Plans: A Simpler Approach; Outlook On Compensation And Benefits,'' *Personnel* (June 1988):30, 34–35; J. Freiden, ''Getting Your Flexible Benefits Program Under Way,'' *Business and Health* (Oct. 1989):44, 46–47.

10. Joint Economic Committee, ''Health Care Briefing Paper'' presented in U.S. House of Representatives, *Oversight Hearing on National Health Care Reform, op. cit.*, pp. 31–32.

11. Joint Economic Committee, ''Health Care Briefing Paper,'' *op. cit.*, p. 11.

12. U.S. House of Representatives, *Oversight Hearing on National Health Care Reform, op. cit.*, p. 62. Heslin was testifying on behalf of the ERISA Industry Committee.

13. Paul Feldstein, *The Politics of Health Legislation: An Economic Perspective* (Ann Arbor, Michigan: Health Administration Press, 1988); Paul Feldstein, ''Why the United States Has Not Had National Health Insurance'' in Robert Huefner and Margaret Battin, eds., *Changing to National Health Care: Ethical and Policy Issues* (Salt Lake City, Utah: University of Utah Press, 1992):51–71.

14. John Motley, III, ''Small Business Access to Affordable Health Care and Health Insurance,'' included in the U.S. House of Representatives, *Long-Term Strategies For Health Care*, Hearings Before the Committee on Ways and Means, House of Representatives, Serial 102–33, 102d Cong., 1st Sess., April 16–17, 23–25, 1991 (Washington, D.C.: U.S. Government Printing Office, 1992), pp. 599–613.

15. John Motley, III, "Small Business Access to Affordable Health Care and Health Insurance," *op. cit.*, p. 601.

16. U.S. Dept. of Labor, Fiduciary Standards Employee Retirement Income Security Act (Washington: Labor-Management Services Administration, 1989).

17. "Consolidated Omnibus Budget Reconciliation Act of 1985 (Public Law 99–272)," *Health Care Financing Review* (Spring 1987):95–115; The Omnibus Budget Reconciliation Act of 1989 (OBRA), P.L. 101–239, was signed into law on December 19, 1989, and made a number of important changes in COBRA.

18. John Motley, III, "Small Business Access to Affordable Health Care and Health Insurance," *op. cit.*, p. 604.

Part IV

National Policy and Strategies

11

Other National Models

When there is a debate about national health care, especially about universal or single payer coverage, it is usually predictable that one of the debating parties will bring up the subject of the Canadian, United Kingdom, or German universal health care systems. In order to set the stage for formulating U.S. national health care strategy, it is necessary to briefly summarize the major characteristics of those systems in order to show that our economy, our form of government, and our democratic and competitive business environment are not consistent with their models of nationalized health care.[1]

CANADIAN MEDICAL CARE

Carol Sakala is careful to distinguish the United States health care proposals from the Canadian and British *medical* care systems.[2] Sakala argues that the universal systems proposed and discussed in the United States encompass much more than medical care, that they "have a broader vision—of a program that, along with medical care, places considerable emphasis on prevention through attention to occupational and environmental exposures; economic security; education; housing; tobacco, alcohol, and injury policies; and other major determinants of health status."[3]

Within the span of just this short passage, Sakala pinpoints the exact difference between what the United States Congress is trying to accomplish versus what the socialized welfare countries have implemented.

There is an enormous difference between the national objectives of medical care versus those of what we commonly refer to as "health care." One could go as far as to suggest that the United States really wants a comprehensive overhaul of the whole medical and health care infrastructure, an all-encompassing concept which includes environmental linkages.

It was not until after World War II, in 1949, that the British North America Act set up the provinces as autonomous units and made medical care a provincial responsibility.[4] After several years of experience with the Saskatchewan, Alberta, Ontario, and Quebec program legislation, 1964–1965 was a watershed period for medical care in the form of the Royal Commission on Health Services Report, the Hall Commission, leading to the Medical Care Act or Medicare. From 1969 to 1972 the Canadian Medicare programs were established throughout all provinces and territories of Canada.[5]

The Canadian system of medical care differs from the health care system in the United States in several respects. With the competitive system of health care in the United States, a large proportion of the health care expenditures are borne by the employer and through private individual insurance. A major difference between the two systems, however, is in the public expenditures sector. Figure 11.1 presents a contrast of the public health expenditures as a percentage of total health expenditures for both Canada and the United States for the period from 1970 through 1989. Notice that in about 1980, the United States' public health expenditures were about 42 percent of total health expenditures, and remained so through 1989. Canada's public health expenditures as a percentage of total health expenditures remained at about 75 percent from 1980 through 1989. Canada's percentages are about 1.8 times those of the United States, yet it has not yet been shown that the quality of Canada's medical care is superior to that in the United States.[6]

When one compares the total health expenditures as a percentage of gross domestic product, as in Figure 11.2, it is obvious that the United States is devoting a larger share of its gross domestic product to medical care and health services than is Canada. For example, Figure 11.2 indicates that Canada spent about 7.1 percent of its gross domestic product on medical care in 1970 and had stabilized out at about 8.7 percent by 1989. In the United States, by contrast, Figure 11.2 indicates that in 1970 health and medical care accounted for 7.4 percent of gross domestic product, and by 1989 the figure had accelerated to 11.8 percent of gross domestic product.

Figure 11.1 Public Health Expenditures as Percentage of Total Health Expenditures

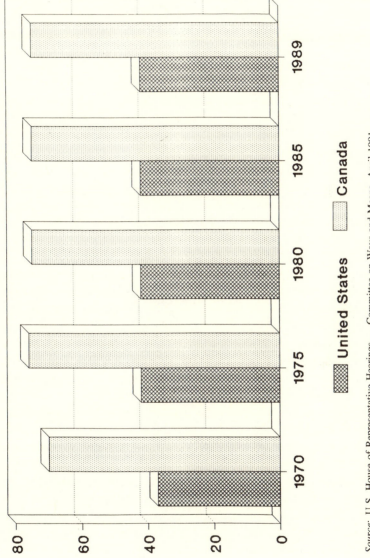

Source: U.S. House of Representative Hearings — Committee on Ways and Means, April 1991, p. 98.

Figure 11.2 Total Health Expenditures as a Percentage of Gross Domestic Product

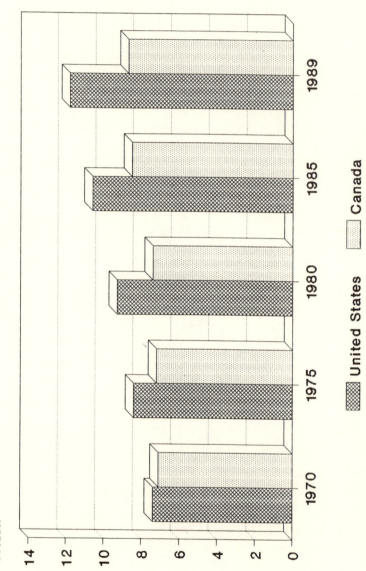

Source: U.S. House of Representatives Hearings — Committee on Ways and Means, April, 1991, p. 100.

The Canadian Assistance Plan has been slow to introduce the latest technology like CT scan and MRI diagnostic equipment throughout the provinces. Both proliferate in the health care networks in America, even in smaller, non-metropolitan areas. Perhaps the difference in ancillary or health care environmental services and the modern technology are the partial cause of the per capita health spending in the United States versus Canada as shown in Figure 11.3.

Figure 11.3 indicates that the United States spent about $2,354 per capita for health care as compared to the $1,683 in Canada. Canada practiced cost containment measures after a number of years of testing varying levels of federal-provincial financing. The Canada Health Act of 1984 also consolidated previous national health insurance laws in order to reform the fee for service practices of the physicians—the physicians are usually salaried employees of the provinces. As Roemer describes the reforms in 1984:

> The conditions stipulated in the two original laws for provincial receipt of federal allotments were also tightened in 1984: (a) the program must be administered by a public authority accountable to the provincial government; (b) the program must cover all necessary hospital and medical care and surgical-dental services rendered in hospitals; (c) 100 percent of the provincial residents must be entitled to insured services; and (d) reasonable access to insured services must not be impeded directly or indirectly by charger or other mechanisms.[7]

Notice that the reforms above did not mention the spectrum of health care services surrounding strict medical care that Americans take for granted. The Canadian system of medical care is analogous to the old time country store—it has most, maybe all, of the bare essentials, but very little, if any, of the ancillary products that complement the basic essentials.[8]

UNITED KINGDOM MEDICAL CARE

There are literally hundreds of studies regarding the state of medical care in the United Kingdom, but there is none which describes that system in more succinct terms than the short description offered by Litman and Robins. They describe the United Kingdom system thusly:

> The basic level would provide reasonably good access to primary care, for the full range of illnesses, with general practitioners as gatekeepers,

Figure 11.3 Per Capita Health Spending in the United States and Canada, 1989

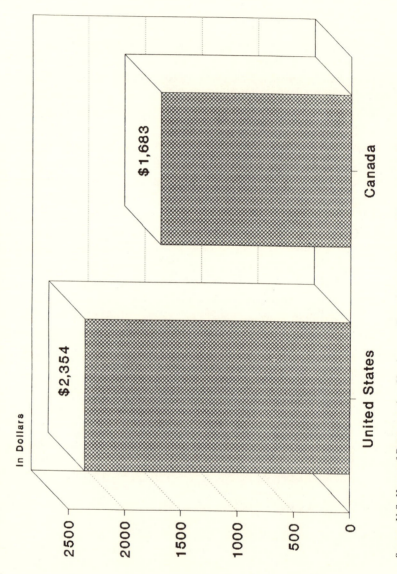

In Dollars

$2,354

$1,683

United States

Canada

2500
2000
1500
1000
500
0

Source: U.S. House of Representatives Hearings — Committee on Ways and Means, April 1991, p. 103.

and quick access to hospitals for acute and emergency care. There might be, however, hemming and hawing on the part of the primary physicians to facilitate quick access or access at all for elective surgery and for medical conditions, treatment for which can be delayed to see how they turn out. This is the United Kingdom Model . . .[9]

The medical care system in the United Kingdom has been called the "most centralized health care system among the advanced industrial nations."[10] Their system employs the capitation method of payment to physicians and a fee-for-service method of payment for specialists. What makes the system in the United Kingdom so interesting is that many of the tough medical alternatives are decided by the physician for the good of the nation. As Francis puts it:

British medicine has brought to health care decision making a social utilitarianism—that is, advice against certain procedures on grounds of the general good rather than the condition and desire of the patient. Older patients may be advised against major surgery on the grounds that they have relatively few productive years remaining, and younger patients might receive a specific procedure on grounds of greater social utility.[11]

This is a very interesting social philosophy, especially for the United States, where good health care and elective procedures are thought to be social "rights." Citizens of the United States may be shocked to find out just how many countries share the philosophy just cited for the United Kingdom.[12] The United Kingdom model has not been cited by many members of Congress as a model that should be used as a pattern for American health care. This is probably because the United Kingdom has maintained the current system essentially since the end of World War II. The current form of the Canadian system has been in place only a few years.

GERMAN SOCIALIZED MEDICAL CARE

It is argued, and probably with some justification, that competition in the health care delivery network may have perverse effects on the distribution of medical care and health care services. It is true that the richer areas in the United States provide better health care services—education, preventive medicine, specialized medicine, and trauma centers. It is also plausible to argue that centralized planning of health care services at all levels of health care will enable a system to distribute health care resources more efficiently and with more equity.

Germany has one of the most elaborate networks of children's creches (nurseries) in the world. Over two-thirds of children under three years of age were enrolled in a creche in Germany. Children also get an allowance through the German social security system. Shortly after World War II, Germany obtained financing from a network of private and governmental funds. Over the years this became more centralized. Roemer describes the current system thusly:

> Now there is a flat 10 percent insurance tax on all wages, shared by the workers and the enterprises, up to a maximum of $24 per month. This is used to finance all benefits (old-age pensions, disability compensation, etc.), including health care. There is also a substantial subsidy from general governmental revenues. Trade unions perform some of the administrative functions. Every GDR resident is entitled to the same service, through the network of polyclinics and hospitals.[13]

The flat tax on wages is now being proposed in the United States Congress, that is, the "pay-or-play" plans are calling for either a 7 percent or 9 percent tax on wages to be paid by the employer if that employer does not offer a federally approved health care plan.

Since virtually every phase of health care in Germany is centrally controlled and planned by the government, there is little or no room for market dynamics or personal physicians to have expressions of entrepreneurship. Physicians are salaried by the GDR, but some private activity can be found in the manufacture of pharmaceuticals, education of health care personnel, and the provision of health care to industrial workers.[14]

There is a superstructure of private practice available to high-incomed Germans. They may elect a private insurance fund in lieu of the "sickness funds," but once they elect to leave a sickness fund for a private insurance carrier, they are not allowed to return to any of the sickness funds. These sickness funds are the health care payers and negotiate with the health care providers for hospitalization costs and fee schedules. Even retired persons have deductions from their retirement checks for these sickness funds. It would be safe to say that the German model could not be implemented easily in the United States in the foreseeable future.[15]

POLICY AND STRATEGY IMPLICATIONS

It is clear that the American health care system is closer to the Canadian system than it is to that of the United Kingdom or of Germany. The United Kingdom and Germany have restrictive systems in which health care ancillary and elective services are not included in the basic health care delivery network. In the Canadian system, there is room for a fee-for-service practice to co-exist with the mandated basic national care. The philosophy of care is altogether different in Europe than in the United States and Canada.

The data in Figure 11.4 dramatize the difference in the philosophy among the United Kingdom (with $836 per capita spending), Germany (with $1,232), Canada (with $1,683), and the United States (with $2,354). The United Kingdom has universal coverage, but the "gatekeeper" physician has powerful authority to allocate "specialist" services to those who need them. Germany, with approximately 50 percent higher expenditures per capita, has basic universal care, but it also has a massive nursery (creche) child care program that has added administrative and overhead costs. The Canadian expenditures, double that of the United Kingdom, include more liberal elective measures and have technology that far exceeds that in the United Kingdom.[16]

The per capita health care spending reflected in Figure 11.4 is a clear indication that very basic health care packages with very strict limitations on access and coverage can be made universally available at far less cost than is the experience in the United States. The demand for comprehensive medical and health care with the very latest in technology is the costly element in the provision of massive health care. If Americans are trying to maintain a "Cadillac and champagne taste on a beer budget tax contribution," health care costs in the United States will continue to escalate and there will be increasing gaps in health care for most of the population and for all of the uninsured population.

The strategy for health care in the United States must have a sharper focus regarding:

1. What constitutes a basic level of health care?
2. What contribution do the workers make toward their own health care and that of the non-workers?
3. Should the provision of health care benefits be the concern of employers?

Figure 11.4 Per Capita Health Spending in United Kingdom, Germany, Canada, and the United States, 1989

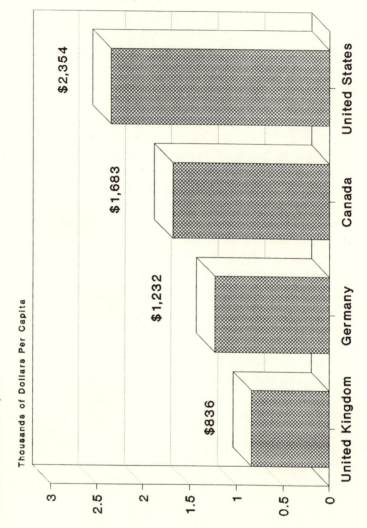

Thousands of Dollars Per Capita

$836 $1,232 $1,683 $2,354

United Kingdom   Germany   Canada   United States

3   2.5   2   1.5   1   0.5   0

Source: U.S. House of Representatives Hearings — Committee on Ways and Means, April 1991, p. 103.

4. To what extent should elective, experimental, and "heroic" measures be covered by private sector plans?
5. How can health care services and resources be more efficiently allocated to minimize cost shifting resulting from uncompensated and undercompensated care?
6. Can we continue to have a private/public partnership in the financing and provision of health care?

The list could contain many times the number of questions posed above, but the questions indicate the kinds of issues that have not been solved or explicitly addressed by Congress in any of the legislative measures presented in the previous chapters. From the U.S. House of Representatives and U.S. Senate bills discussed earlier, it is obvious that the Democrats want to have some kind of universal health care. The Republicans and private foundations want market reform and prefer to have a market-driven health care system. Since they represent the two dominant philosophies in Congress, there must be some common position that will allow the underlying element separating them—*financing, or who will pay*—to be worked out. Up to this point in time, the Democratic universal health care proposals include very heavy dependence on contributions from employers, thus placing them at odds with business and industry. The "pay-or-play" plans should really be called the "*pay-or-pay*" plans, since they require the employers to either *pay* the government for a state-run plan or *pay* for a plan to cover all employees and their families on their own initiative.

In the next chapter we will discuss some of the elements of health care rationing before we develop a national health care plan in the fifth part of this book. In the foreword to the author's earlier book on health care, *Mandated Health Care: Issues and Strategies*, Thomas Curtis remarked, "The author suggests in his review of the literature and from his own experience and reasoning that some rationing is inevitable. I don't totally agree. There are ample means (money) and resources to meet the needs of the 15 percent who cannot afford any health care."[17]

He is right. There are enough resources to provide all persons with basic health care, but the sticking point seems to turn on who pays, how it is delivered, and how resources are allocated among competing demands of differing priorities.

NOTES

1. One of the very best sources for cross-country comparisons is given in Milton Roemer, *National Health Systems of the World* (New York: Oxford University Press, 1991). This source covers virtually every country in the world.

2. Carol Sakala, "The Development of National Medical Care Programs in the United Kingdom and Canada: Applicability to Current Conditions in the United States," *Journal of Health Politics, Policy and Law* (Winter 1990):709–753.

3. Carol Sakala, "The Development of National Medical Care Programs . . . ," *op. cit.*, pp. 717–718.

4. Milton Roemer, *National Health Systems of the World, op. cit.*, p.161. See also Malcolm Taylor, *Health Insurance and Canadian Public Policy: The Seven Decisions That Created the Canadian Health Insurance System* (Montreal: McGill-Queen's University Press, 1978) and Malcolm Taylor, *Health Insurance and Canadian Public Policy: The Seven Decisions That Created the Canadian Health Insurance System and Their Outcomes* 2d ed. (Toronto: Institute of Public Administration of Canada, 1987). These latter two works are the authoritative works on the Canadian medical care system.

5. A chronology of key events in Canada's development of a national medical care system is given in Table 2 of Carol Sakala, "The Development of National Medical Care Programs . . . ," *op. cit.*, pp. 716–717.

6. Morris Barer and Robert Evans, "Interpreting Canada: Models, Mind-Sets, and Myths," *Health Affairs* (Spring 1992):44–61; Morris Barer, Roger Evans, and Roberta Labelle, "Fee Controls As Cost Control: Tales From The Frozen North," *The Milbank Quarterly* 66:1 (1988):1–64.

7. Milton Roemer, *National Health Systems of the World, op. cit.*, p. 167.

8. Robert Evans et al., "Controlling Health Expenditures—The Canadian Reality," *New England Journal of Medicine* (2 March 1989):571–577; Robert Evans, *Strained Mercy: The Economics of Canadian Health Care* (Toronto: Butterworth, 1984); Bertha Bryant, "Issues on the Distribution of Health Care: Some Lessons from Canada," *Public Health Reports* (September-October 1981):442–447; Malcolm Taylor, *Health Insurance and Canadian Public Policy: The Seven Decisions That Created the Canadian Health Insurance System and Their Outcomes* 2d ed., *op. cit.*; and Morris Barer and Robert Evans, "Interpreting Canada: Models, Mind-Sets, and Myths," *Health Affairs, op cit.*

9. Theodore Litman and Leonard Robins, *Health Politics and Policy*, 2nd ed. (New York: Delmar Publishers, 1991), p. 80.

10. John Francis, "Lessons from Abroad in Assessing National Health Care Systems: Ethics and Decision Making" in Robert Huefner and Margaret Battin, eds., *Changing to National Health Care: Ethical and Policy Issues* (Salt Lake City, Utah: University of Utah Press, 1992):99.

11. John Francis, *ibid.*, p. 99.

12. Christopher Ham, *Health Policy in Britain: The Politics and Organization of the National Health Service* (London: Macmillan, 1985); William Schwartz and Henry Aaron, "Rationing Hospital Care: Lessons from Britain," *New England Journal of Medicine* (5 January 1984):52–56; John Lister, "The Politics of Medicine in Britain and the United States," *New England Journal of Medicine* (17 July 1986):168–173; John Lister, "Pro-

posals for Reform of the British National Health Service,'' *New England Journal of Medicine* (30 March 1989):877–880.

13. Milton Roemer, *National Health Systems of the World, op. cit.*, p. 262.

14. William Glaser, ''Lessons from Germany: Some Reflections Occasioned by Schulenberg's Report,'' *Journal of Health Politics, Policy and Law* (Summer 1983):352–365; Christa Altenstetter, ''An End to a Consensus on Health Care in the Federal Republic of Germany?'' *Journal of Health Politics, Policy and Law* (Fall 1987):505–536; Donald Light et al., ''Social Medicine vs. Professional Dominance: The German Experience,'' *American Journal of Public Health* (January 1986):78–83.

15. Paul Godt, ''Confrontation, Consent and Corporatism: State Strategies and the Medical Profession in France, Great Britain, and West Germany,'' *Journal of Health Politics, Policy and Law* (Fall 1987):459–480.

16. Geoffrey Weller, ''Common Problems, Alternative Solutions: A Comparison of the Canadian and American Health Systems,'' *Policy Studies Journal* (June 1986):604–620; Robert Evans et al., ''Controlling Health Expenditures—The Canadian Reality,'' *New England Journal of Medicine, op. cit.*, passim.

17. Donald Westerfield, *Mandated Health Care: Issues and Strategies* (New York: Praeger, 1991), p. xii.

12

Rationing Policies and Strategies

The previous chapter ended with a statement that we would not need to ration health care if we were willing to devote enough of our existing resources to solve the problem. That statement would be true if we all had a common perception of the "health care problem" and what it encompasses. Congress has not been able to formulate an acceptable state of the nature or scope of the health care problem. Special interests, business and industry, the underclass, the health care payers and providers, the insurers, and every other major stakeholder group has a different perception of the health care problem.[1] Lacking a clear consensus view of the problem, it would seem reasonable to argue that everyone should be entitled to at least some basic level of health care.

How do we handle the problem of persons with incurable diseases, or underweight babies that are predicted to live no more than a few weeks or months, or those with terminal illnesses, or those who need organ transplants, or those in persistent vegetative (so-called "brain dead") conditions? These problems require remedies that go beyond a basic level of care. The previous chapter indicated that in the United Kingdom medical care above some basic level may go unprovided in given circumstances.[2] Can Americans cope with making the decisions required to give more medical care to some and less to others? Almost everyone would agree that rationing in America is a certainty, as it is in every other country. Unlimited access and care for everyone is improbable and imprudent.[3]

"HORIZONTAL" VERSUS "VERTICAL" CARE

The concept of "horizontal" care implies that a person must be in a horizontal position to obtain care, that is, the person must be sick enough to not be ambulatory to obtain care. This is emergency or acute care. Surely this level of care should be guaranteed to everyone.[4] What about horizontal, but long-term or catastrophic? In the United Kingdom, this is a case for a bit more consideration. The age and productivity of the patient would have to be integrated into the decision-making procedure for these cases.[5]

We get the impression from many of the bills from the United States Congress discussed throughout chapters 5 through 7 of this book that "horizontal" acute and emergency care will be provided to most persons in the basic package. How much of the "vertical" care will be provided based on those same proposed bills is not clear. What is not generally known by the nonelderly population, those under age 65 years of age, is that Medicare has limits on its coverage. Many recipients of Medicare must buy "Medigap" insurance to cover a whole spectrum of health care drugs, aids, appliances, and services. Even those items just listed for the "horizontal" patients may not be totally covered by the existing Medicare coverage.

Some areas of "vertical" care are covered—things such as well baby care, pregnant woman care, certain female disease detection and prevention services, and a limited list of social and psychological services are provided as parts of a "basic" health care package.[6] The American concept of all-around care, not just medical care, means that the expectations of the wider range of health care demanded by most Americans cannot be satisfied without tremendous increases in health care expenditures and an extremely liberal health care plan.

CHRONIC AND CATASTROPHIC CASES

This category of persons is responsible for the greatest burden placed on the health care system. In earlier sections it was estimated that at least 90 percent of the health care expenditures in America are caused by 10 percent of the population. Typically, the extremely old and the extremely young compose the major part of this category of persons. Underweight babies with short life expectancies, some born at a birth weight of less than 2 pounds, and the chronically ill elderly use up a significant proportion of our health care resources. Both of these categories of persons are probably categorized in the "horizontal" group. They often require around-the-clock professional attention, require special monitoring equipment, may require life-sustaining equipment and measures, and often involve significant legal problems. Medicare and Medicaid coverage is not set up for these categories of persons.

With the passage of the Tax Equity and Fiscal Responsibility Act of 1982 (TEFRA) and the Deficit Reduction Act of 1984 (DEFRA), Medicare is made a *secondary* payer instead of a *primary* payer for those *workers and their spouses* who are aged 65 through 69 years. Currently, employers must provide health care coverage for the spouses despite the chronic and/or catastrophic nature of the illness of a spouse, even though the spouse does not contribute to the productivity of the employer.[7]

The health care market reforms examined in chapter 7 of this book are "spotty" regarding their coverages of the chronically ill and those with catastrophic illnesses. The trend in employer plans, absent those proposed in the previous chapters, is to place caps on the total dollars per episode or for the lifetime of an employee. Additionally, the plans specifically limit or even do not cover certain illnesses or conditions that are expected to be financial liabilities within the covered group.

The universal plans, with exceptions, typically employ a cost shifting strategy and let the states or employers figure out what will be done with the chronic and catastrophic cases. What might prove to be less costly to the government and what might provide the kind of coverage needed by this very desperate group is to expand Medicaid to cover all chronic and catastrophic cases for families with incomes below 200 percent of the poverty level and to have Medicare be first payer for all chronic and catastrophic cases at or above age 65.[8] The federal government could negotiate with private firms to provide "pool coverage" for cases that look like they will require catastrophic expenditures.

LONG-TERM CARE

David Holzman wrote an article titled "Endless Care with Costs to Match," which many believe to be the core of the issue of long-term care.[9] Both Medicaid and Medicare break down when it comes to providing care over an extended period. Typically, business and industry have avoided the long-term care issue. Moreover, the trend for the last half of the eighties and the first part of the nineties is to decrease or outright eliminate health care benefits for retirees, especially if the language of the company health care plan will permit it.[10]

The strategy on the part of government and employers with respect to long-term care, therefore, has been to shift the costs to someone else or to not address the problem at all. Of the bills from Congress discussed in chapters 5 through 7 of this book, some examples of those that explicitly discuss long-term care are H.R. 8—Comprehensive Health Care Act (Oakar), S. 1446—Health USA Act of 1991 (Kerrey), and H.R. 3535—USHealth Program Act of 1991 (Roybal).[11] Part of the reason why Congress is reticent to deal with the long-term care issue is the debacle associated with the Medicare Catastrophic Coverage Act of 1988, Public Law 100–360, which was repealed in late 1989. Congress was united to pass such an act based on pressure from special interest groups representing elders. When that group found out that they would actually have to pay a surcharge for the benefits, they successfully lobbied Congress to repeal it.[12]

That strategy by elder special interest groups, especially the American Association of Retired Persons (AARP) and the National Committee to Preserve Social Security and Medicare, put a sour taste in the mouth of Congress for both catastrophic coverage as well as long-term care coverage for elders. The death of Representative Claude Pepper, the champion of causes for the elderly and retired persons, additionally had its impact on the coalition in Congress, especially the House of Representatives, which had been the progenitor of much of the legislation for the elderly.

POOR, NEAR POOR, AND THE MEDICALLY INDIGENT

As mentioned earlier in this chapter, the elderly have typically enjoyed a very strong lobby in Congress, as have the pregnant women and mothers with tiny infants. The portion of the American population which "fell through the cracks" is what many refer to as the "underclass," consisting of the poor, the near poor, and the medically indigent.[13] The definitions of poor and near poor are tenuous, especially to economists who study "aid in kind," "entitlements," and "transfers" to the category of persons who are typically and non-technically called "poor." Whoever they are, they do not receive the kind of preventive health care and regular attention that persons in that category typically receive.[14]

What makes this underclass so difficult to deal with is the fact that some persons in this category tend to fluctuate in and out of this category, while some are permanently there with no relief. They typically work part-time or not at all—often not due to their own choice. This situation is compounded by stigma and sometimes social prejudice. What is more important, they are the least represented by special interests in Congress and there are few advocacy resources to carry their message to the various legislative committees. Any strategy for comprehensive coverage or even health care reform should include the extension of Medicaid benefits to this underclass. A "means test" could be required to determine who participates in the plan free of charge and who has the ability to pay and, therefore, should pay.[15]

Ideally, health care benefits for the underclass should not be tied in any way to the employer. This permits portability and ensures that there is continuity of coverage when the marginal worker is temporarily out of work (or in work, as the case may be). Medically indigent persons should be covered by at least a basic plan with all premiums waived, unless that person has an income source that places the person above 200 percent of the poverty level or some level determined to be both practical and equitable.[16]

MANAGED CARE

When health care services are provided to any segment of the population without cost or copayment, there is a tendency for the recipients to use the services more frequently and with more intensity than might be necessary or appropriate. Having a managed care program coupled with a primary care physician who is the continuing and initial entry point into the health care delivery system could help to minimize such occurrences. Mr. J. B. Silvers of the Prospective Payment Assessment Commission addresses this problem in his testimony before the U.S. House of Representatives Long-Term Strategies for Health Care Hearings:

Hospitals are increasing the types and amounts of services furnished to all patients regardless of whether they are more complex or severely ill. We refer to this factor as "intensity" of services. Changes in the intensity of patient care account for 1.8 percentage points per year, or 20 percent of the annual increase in hospital costs per case. This intensity increase includes two components: increase due to technologic advancements and increase due to the expanded use of existing technologies and services. We estimate that about one-third of the annual cost increases from intensity is due to major new advances and two-thirds is due to increased use of established tests and procedures.[17]

A program of managed care for major user groups could act as a cost containment measure and could also be used to measure the quality of care delivered and received by those within the major user groups. The same argument could be made regarding implementing managed care in both the Medicare and Medicaid programs, as recommended by the Business Roundtable.[18] It should be pointed out that there is a major effort among legislators to eliminate the use of managed care programs in the universal coverage plans. The argument for doing so is that the "gatekeeper" function and the accumulation of information regarding utilization by patient, physician, and by other categories could be used as a method of discrimination at some future time. Most health care analysts believe this argument to be based more on conjecture than actual fact.

In the next chapter we lay the foundation for a national health care plan and strategies for its implementation. Of course, there is still the nagging question regarding whether America is ready for a national plan or just a series of health care reforms.

NOTES

1. American College of Physicians, "Access to Health Care," *Annals of Internal Medicine* 112 (May 1990):642–661; American Hospital Association, *National Health Strategy: A Starting Point for Debate* (Chicago: American Hospital Association, 1991); Richard Brown, "Principles for a National Health Program: A Framework for Analysis and Development," *Milbank Quarterly* 4 (1988):573–617.

2. Theodore Litman and Leonard Robins, *Health Politics and Policy*, 2nd ed. (New York: Delmar Publishers, 1991), p. 80.

3. Robert H. Blank, *Rationing Medicine* (New York: Columbia University Press, 1988).

4. Robert Reishauer, Testimony before U.S. House of Representatives, *Long-Term Strategies For Health Care*, Hearings Before the Committee on Ways and Means, House of Representatives, Serial 102–33, 102d Cong., 1st Sess., April 16–17, 23–25, 1991 (Washington, D.C.: U.S. Government Printing Office, 1992), pp. 413–414.

5. Theodore Litman and Leonard Robins, *Health Politics and Policy*, 2nd ed., *op. cit.*, p. 80.

6. U.S. House of Representatives, "Medicare Universal Coverage Expansion Act of 1991," H.R. 1777, 102d Cong., 1st Sess., *Congressional Record—Extension of Remarks* (16 April 1991):E1261-E1262; U.S. House of Representatives, "Universal Health Care Act of 1991," H.R. 1300, 102d Cong., 2nd Sess. (Washington, D.C.: U.S. Government Printing Office, 1992); U.S. House of Representatives, "Comprehensive Health Care for All Americans Act" (Claude Pepper Comprehensive Health Care Act), H.R. 8, 102d Cong., 1st Sess. (Washington, D.C.: U.S. Government Printing Office, 1991). The other bills listed in chapter 5 cover much the same ground.

7. Donald Westerfield, *Mandated Health Care: Issues and Strategies* (New York: Praeger, 1991), pp. 26–27; Donald Westerfield and Paul Wilson, "Employers and the

Medicare Secondary Payer: IRS/SSA/HCFA Data Match Project,'' *Proceedings of the Business and Health Administration Association* (March 1992):127–130.

8. John Holahan and Sheila Zedlewski, ''Insuring Low-Income Americans Through Medicaid Expansion,'' Urban Institute Working Paper No. 3836–02 (December 1989); Susan Garland, ed., ''The Torpedo That Slammed Into Catastrophic Health Care,'' *Business Week* (23 Oct. 1989):70; J. W. Fossett, J. A. Peterson, and M. C. Ring, ''Public Sector Primary Care And Medicaid: Trading Accessibility For Mainstreaming,'' *Journal Of Health Politics, Policy And Law* 14 (Fall 1989):309–325.

9. David Holzman, ''Endless Care With Costs To Match,'' *Insight* (Dec.–Jan. 1987):44–46.

10. ''Assessing the Future of Long-Term Care,'' *Healthspan* (Mar. 1988):6–15; Jay Boekhoff and Robert Dobson, ''The Long Term Care Insurance Challenge,'' *Emphasis* (Oct. 1987):6–8; A. E. Benjamin, ''Long-term Care And AIDS: Perspectives From Experience With The Elderly,'' *The Milbank Quarterly* 66:3 (1988):415–443; Anita Bruzzese, ''Companies Cut Retiree Benefits,'' *Employee Benefit News* Vol. 1 (Apr. 1987):1, 36.

11. U.S. House of Representatives, ''Comprehensive Health Care for All Americans Act'' (Claude Pepper Comprehensive Health Care Act), H.R. 8, 102d Cong., 1st Sess. (Washington, D.C.: U.S. Government Printing Office, 1991); U.S. Senate. ''Health USA Act of 1991,'' S. 1446, 102d Cong., 1st Sess. (Washington, D.C.: U.S. Government Printing Office, 1991); U.S. House of Representatives, ''USHealth Program Act of 1991,'' H.R. 3535, 102d Cong., 2d Sess. (Washington, D.C.: U.S. Government Printing Office, 1992).

12. Donald Westerfield, *Mandated Health Care: Issues and Strategies, op. cit.*, pp. 30–31.

13. John Holahan and Sheila Zedlewski, ''Insuring Low-Income Americans Through Medicaid Expansion,'' Urban Institute Working Paper No. 3836–02 (December 1989); ''Health Care Coverage by Age, Sex, Race, and Family Income: United States, 1986,'' *Medical Benefits* (31 Oct. 1987):3–4; Lucy Johns and Gerald Adler, ''Evaluation Of Recent Changes In Medicaid,'' *Health Affairs* (Spring 1989):171–181.

14. Karen Davis and Cathy Schoen, *Health and the War on Poverty: A Ten-Year Appraisal* (Washington, D.C.: The Brookings Institution, 1978).

15. L. R. Churchill, *Rationing Health Care In America: Perceptions And Principles Of Justice* (Notre Dame: University of Notre Dame Press, 1987).

16. Jack Meyer, ed., *Market Reforms in Health Care: Current Issues, New Directions, Strategic Decisions* (Washington, D.C.: American Enterprise Institute for Public Policy Research, 1983); Stephen Long and Jack Rogers, ''The Effects of Being Uninsured on Health Care Service Use Estimates from the Survey of Income and Program Participation,'' *Survey of Income and Program Participation (SIPP) Working Paper No. 9012* (Washington, D.C.: Bureau of the Census, 1990).

17. Testimony of J. B. Silvers before the U.S. House of Representatives, *Long-Term Strategies For Health Care, op. cit.*, p. 210.

18. Testimony of Robert C. Winters, The Business Roundtable, before the U.S. House of Representatives, *Long-Term Strategies For Health Care, op. cit.*, p. 432.

Part V

A National Health Care Plan

13

Workers Compensation

Before setting out the characteristics of a national plan in the following chapter, it is necessary to address a portion of the current health care system which has been hidden from the view of the general public. The Workers Compensation system, which includes a major health care expenditure by business and industry, has been the "sacred cow" of states and has been impervious to federal legislative attempts to reform it. Young and Polakoff observe that:

> Medical care, for example, is a substantial component of workers' compensation costs, and medical costs are increasing in workers' compensation at least as fast, and probably faster, than in other medical care delivery systems . . . workers' compensation costs have escalated significantly. Costs have increased much faster than wages, up from 1.14% of payroll in 1972 to 2.06% in 1987. The cost per employee increased from $93 in 1972 to $430 in 1987. Total workers' compensation costs increased during this period from $5.8 billion to $38 billion.[1]

What the observation by Young and Polakoff points out is that the Workers Compensation system has become a significant cost to employers when superimposed upon already existing employee benefit costs, and, as Figures 13.1 and 13.2 point out, the rate of growth of both the costs per employee and the costs in billions of dollars, respectively, between 1972 and 1987 have national significance. The "per employee" costs increased over 4.6 times its 1972 value by 1987, while the total costs for

Figure 13.1 Workers Compensation Costs Per Employee

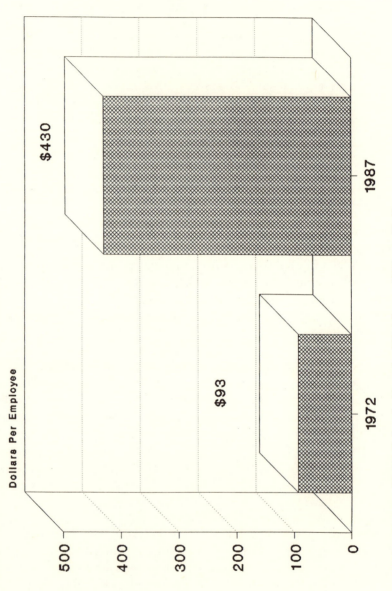

Dollars Per Employee

$430

$93

1987

1972

500

400

300

200

100

0

Source: Young and Polakoff, Benefits Quarterly, (Third Quarter 1992), pp. 56–65.

Figure 13.2 Total Workers Compensation Costs

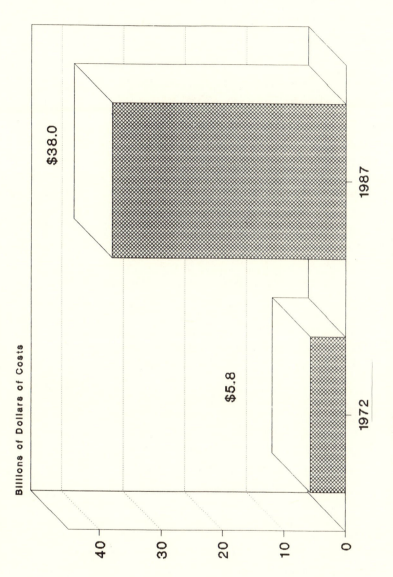

Billions of Dollars of Costs

$38.0

$5.8

1987

1972

40

30

20

10

0

Source: Young and Polakoff, Benefits Quarterly, (Third Quarter 1992), pp. 56–65.

Workers Compensation, in billions of dollars, grew 6.55 times its 1972 value by 1987. Since a major component of these costs are medical costs, there is concern that these costs will spiral in a fashion similar to the spiral in medical costs in the last decade.

STATE SYSTEM "OUT OF CONTROL"

All 50 states have a Workers Compensation program that is autonomous from other state programs as well as from federal programs.[2] Corporate and small business managers indicate that the system costs have gotten completely out of control. The mast of an article by Jerry Miccolis, analyzing the Workers Compensation system, states, "The State of the System—The bad news—according to a comprehensive survey of U.S. employers—is that WC costs are out of control."[3] What is not generally known to the public is that the Workers Compensation system for the most part has

1. No "managed care" program for the medical portion.
2. No copay provisions for medical care and treatment.
3. No deductibles for medical care and treatment.
4. No *lifetime or annual limits on benefits* that an employee may collect.
5. Essentially no control over costs associated with "second injuries," even though they might be only partially job related.
6. Very little control over awards to persons claiming job-related disabilities.
7. Almost no control on amounts spent on disability rehabilitation and occupational rehabilitation.

Managers say that the Workers Compensation system is a virtual "blank check" to physicians and lawyers when there is a job-related accident requiring medical treatment and/or disability rehabilitation. Managers indicate that a covered employee, if given the choice between having the on-the-job injury treated by the regular employee health plan or Workers Compensation, will choose the Workers Compensation alternative because there are no deductibles, no copay, no limits, and very little resistance to large awards. This is one reason why the Workers Compensation rates are so high in high-injury-incidence industries.

SECOND INJURIES

The whole area of "second injuries" is a very difficult legal area, due primarily to the nature of the second injury concept itself. An injury (second injury) may have been inflicted upon a previous injury (first injury, which might not have been work related) in such a manner as to result in disability. Even if the first and second injuries were not work related, occupational therapy may be required to restore the employee to some productive capacity. Whether and to what extent second injuries are covered varies from state to state. Examples from the *1990 Analysis of Workers Compensation Laws* of second injuries which are covered under the Workers Compensation provisions for selected states are

1. Arizona—"Second injury which added to a pre-existing work-related disability or a pre-existing physical impairment not industrially related (25 types of handicaps as listed by statute) results in disability for work."
2. California—"Second permanent partial injury which added to pre-existing permanent partial disability results in 70 percent or more permanent disability. Second injury must account for 35 percent."
3. Indiana—"Second injury involving loss or loss of use of hand, arm, foot, leg, or eye which added to pre-existing loss or loss of use of member results in permanent total disability."
4. Maryland—"Second injury which combined with a pre-existing permanent impairment due to accident, disease, or cogenital condition results in a greater combined disability constituting a hindrance to employment."[4]

The examples given above are but four of fifty different versions of the second injuries which are covered by the fifty states. In most cases, the employer has to pay the costs associated with the disability caused by the second injury, even though the first injury might not have been job related. Several of the states pay for the first 104 weeks of disability, and then the remainder of the disability is covered by the state "second injury fund." The second injury funds were set up such that employers pay compensation related primarily to the disability caused by the second injury without regard to the first injury. The fund makes up the difference between the disability benefit the employee receives relating to the combined disability and the disability caused by the second injury alone.

MEDICAL BENEFITS "CARVE OUT"

Would it be reasonable to "carve out" the medical benefits from the Workers Compensation system and transfer the responsibility for that medical care to a national health care system? Carving the medical benefits from the Workers Compensation system would reduce the legal costs involved in medical care required for any injury, job related or not, or occupational disease. The added costs resulting from an industry with an above average incidence of injury or occupational disease could be covered by having the firms in such an industry pay actuarially determined "risk premiums" in accordance with the injury or occupational disease experience of each firm within the industry. In this manner, the safer industries and firms would not be subsidizing the risks of the industries and firms which are inherently high-risk.

Without transferring the medical and health component of Workers Compensation to a national health care system, the fifty states will continue to waste administrative resources in trying to decide which portion of an injury must be handled by which state agency or the employer. Young and Polakoff state the case as:

A considerable amount of effort is expended attempting to keep expenditures within the appropriate program. Health plans try to make sure they do not pay for injuries that should be paid by workers' compensation; the state disability insurance program attempts to recover amounts paid in workers' compensation cases; the state Department of Rehabilitation and the various employment and training programs are careful not to use their resources for persons who should be using workers' compensation. Instead of spending all the administrative resources trying to make sure expenditures for injured and ill workers are placed in the right accounting column, these resources could be used more productively . . .[5]

Such a medical carve out would vitiate the need for a second-injury fund and would preclude the incidence of "adverse selection" strategies which attempt to shift payment from one program to another.

NOTES

1. Casey Young and Phillip Polakoff, "Beyond Workers' Compensation: A New Vision" *Benefits Quarterly* (3rd Quarter 1992):56–65; National Commission on State

Workmen's Compensation Laws, *The Report of the National Commission on State Workmen's Compensation Laws* (Washington, D.C.: U.S. Government Printing Office, 1972).

2. U.S. Chamber of Commerce, *1991 Analysis of Workers Compensation Laws* (Washington, D.C.: U.S. Chamber of Commerce, 1991).

3. Jerry Miccolis, "Workers' Compensation—The State of the System," *Emphasis* (1991/1992):15–17.

4. U.S. Chamber of Commerce, *1990 Analysis of Workers Compensation Laws* (Washington, D.C.: U.S. Chamber of Commerce, 1991), Chart XIII.

5. Casey Young and Phillip Polakoff, "Beyond Workers' Compensation: A New Vision," *Benefits Quarterly*, *op. cit.*, p. 60; see also Insurance Information Institute, *Workers' Compensation Insurance: Protecting America's Workers* (New York: Insurance Information Institute, 1981).

The author is grateful to Paul Wilson, C.P.C.U.-C.E.B.S., for his suggestion that this topic should be considered for inclusion in this work. Other corporate executives have since confirmed the need to formally acknowledge the crisis developing in the Workers Compensation network and have suggested changes needed to reform the Workers Compensation system.

14

Proposed National
Health Care Plan

Throughout the preceding chapters, the major emphasis has been on the legislation proposed in Congress. While other foundation and individual plans have been cited and discussed indirectly, the primary focus has been on the health care proposals that are likely to become the law of the land. As scholars and foundations testify in the hearings before the respective committees in Congress, their philosophies and plan features are then incorporated into the bills that become law. The two major hearings on health care in the Congress have been the *Long-Term Strategies for Health Care* in the U.S. House of Representatives Ways and Means Committee and the *Oversight Hearing on National Health Care Reform* in the U.S. House of Representatives Committee on Education and Labor, the former in the first session of the 102nd Congress and the latter in the second session of the 102nd Congress.[1]

Analyzing the testimony in the hearings just cited confirms the notion that in order to have a national health care system, it must be an underlying premise of that system that *every* American citizen, naturalized citizen, and alien resident should be entitled to basic level or "core" health care benefits. It should also be an underlying premise of that system that everyone who can afford to pay toward those health care benefits should do so. Finally, a major underlying premise of such a national system should be that government alone has the ultimate responsibility for the health and welfare of its citizens and not business or industry.

While the "market reform" proposals have good intentions and will expand coverage to target groups of persons, they really are "employer-based'' reforms that shift costs and responsibility for health care from the government to the employer. A moment's reflection will allow us to recall that health care benefits came into the workplace through ''collective bargaining.'' They were and should be just one more increment of compensation given to employees for their productivity and service. When government mandates benefits on employers, it deliberately increases the firm's costs, increases the firm's product price, and decreases the firm's ability to compete in domestic and foreign markets. More important, however, is the impact on employment—mandated benefits increase unemployment.

Since the ''pay-or-play'' proposals require the employer to provide health care benefits of the type and amount mandated by the federal government or pay the government to provide them, the ''pay-or-play'' proposals should really be called ''pay-or-pay'' proposals. They also are employer mandates and suffer from the deficiencies cited above. They are a cost shifting device which would drive some businesses out of business and heavily burden those small and intermediate sized businesses which might be lucky enough to survive.

The national plan proposed below is based on systems which have been operating for over a quarter of a century and have served millions of Americans well. If the nation really does want national health care, it must be willing to pay the price for it—financially as well as socially. Is it reasonable to expect a consensus on a national health care plan? The mood in Congress has been more receptive to national health care than at any previous time in history. Let us examine the countervailing forces for such a plan.

BIPARTISAN CONSENSUS

The difference of philosophies between the Democrats and the Republicans has been a major impediment to obtaining a consensus on national health care. The Democrats would like to see a universal plan supported and implemented through the nation's employers.[2] The Republicans would like to reform the existing system, but expand access and coverage by lifting some of the burden from employers through tax credits and even the creation of a ''voucher based'' system.[3] The views may be politically divided, but they are not irreconcilable. The political ''sticking point'' is how to finance expanded access.

The experience with the Medicare Catastrophic Coverage Act, for which the elders lobbied so aggressively and against which they lobbied equally as aggressively once they found out that they would have to pay a token amount for it, left a ''bad taste in the mouths'' of the members of Congress who sponsored the legislation and then had to vote to repeal it. What was at the core of this congressional fiasco? *Who pays!* The American experience with entitlements is that those benefitting do not want to pay for anything ''from the government.'' It's just that simple.

In order to obtain a consensus in Congress and with the American people, any national plan must be perceived as

1. Equitable to recipients and payers.
2. Financially stable and affordable.
3. Providing basic, but adequate health care benefits.
4. Involving the absolute minimum of ''red tape'' to obtain benefits and file claims.
5. Universally and continuously accessible.
6. Quality care, with some respect for the dignity of the patients.

Like any list of characteristics, this one could go on and on, but it covers the major concerns of policymakers as well as those who place demands on the health care delivery system. What is really at the heart of the health care delivery system is whether it is ''hassle free'' to both users and payers.

The biggest barrier to congressional consensus may be the killer ''T-word''—taxes in any form. Mentioning taxes in Washington is like the advertisement for E. F. Hutton on television—everyone in the room immediately stops talking and listens. In order to obtain a consensus in Congress, the ''T-word'' should be used with the greatest discretion. This can be done if everyone pays a little . . . and from every reasonable source. Studies abound regarding the threshold for taxes, and they do indicate that almost everyone is willing to have a small tax increase to obtain reasonable health care. The American Medical Association, in testimony before the Ways and Means Committee of the U.S. House of Representatives indicates that:

By a large majority (69%), Americans say the federal government should spend more on the delivery of health care, even if that means an increase in taxes. Still, most of those estimating how much more they would be willing to pay do not want taxes increased by over $100 a year. A majority would like to see federal programs expanded to cover only people not already insured, rather than the establishment of broad-based federal programs to cover all citizens.[4]

Most health care scholars agree that "free" health care would be over-utilized. There must be some cost attached to the use of the health care system, even if the cost per use is ever so slight—perhaps as HMOs charge $3 to $5 for each prescription and $5 to $10 per visit to a physician. The actual amount is less important than the principle that there should be some payment for service by those able to pay. Additionally, there should be some contribution toward the premium by everyone able to pay. Fortunately, these two points are agreed upon by both political parties in Congress.

EMPLOYER MANDATE EXEMPTIONS

A central premise of any workable national health care system must be that the health and welfare of citizens of the United States are the sole responsibility of the United States government and not that of any em-ployer. Whether an employer volunteers to provide health care benefits above any federally provided "core" benefits should depend solely on the discretion of the employer. It should depend on his or her evaluation of whether health care benefits should be included as an increment in the total employee compensation package.

Based on the above premise, all employers would be exempt from federal, state, or local health care benefit mandates. Basic health care benefits would be provided premium free, with restrictions discussed below, through Regional Health Care Centers and would be independent of and autonomous from any voluntary benefits that employers may want to provide. No employer would offer basic or "core" benefits, since these benefits would be obtained from and the responsibility of the federal "single payer" system. If any employer voluntarily offered supplemental health care benefits above and beyond the governmental "core" benefits, the Internal Revenue Service would allow that employer a 100 percent tax deduction for the costs associated with such a voluntary program up to an amount that does not exceed 75 percent of the cost of the government "core" benefits.

Government mandates such as COBRA,[5] TEFRA,[6] and DEFRA,[7] and those related (and subsequently amended) sections of ERISA[8] relating to an employer's providing health care benefits should be repealed, with no replacement. These acts have been barriers to the voluntary provision of health care benefits by small employers, due to their inflexibility and inappropriateness for spreading actuarial risks and costs across a reasonably-sized exposure group.

FLOOR FOR "HORIZONTAL" CASES

The basic health care package provided should be considered a floor of basic medical care and treatment, or "core" benefits, which provides free emergency medical treatment and services to all American citizens or naturalized citizens below 100 percent of the poverty level through the expansion of a Medicaid-type program or through the expansion of Medicaid itself, without the Medicaid restrictions on access. This would include free ambulatory emergency medical treatment and services, but would not include treatment and services associated with catastrophic or chronic symptoms associated with conditions or illnesses such as or requiring organ transplants, dialysis, cancer, alcohol and drug addiction, mental illness, and "heroic" or experimental medicine. Treatment associated with such catastrophic and chronic symptoms as listed above would be covered under "add-on" policies offered through "high-risk pools" and/or funded by private foundations. The state could implement and fund such a high-risk pool if private industry could not or would not set up such an arrangement.

The "gatekeeper" or "primary physician" would control excessive treatment and access to specialists required under the basic plan. Managed care would be mandatory as a cost containment measure and to provide a method of quality assurance.

CAPITATED DIAGNOSIS RELATED GROUPS (DRGS)

The National Association of Children's Hospitals and Related Institutions testified before the U.S. House of Representatives that

Medicare's DRG-based prospective payment system is inappropriate for pediatric hospital care for several reasons:

• Medicare DRGs (diagnosis related groups)—as a method of case-mix classification—do not distinguish sufficiently among the resource demands of treating different pediatric diagnoses.[9]

The current system of Diagnosis Related Groups (DRGs) or International Classification of Diseases (ICD9s) should be expanded to include the whole spectrum of pediatric, geriatric, and other resource needs commonly and routinely experienced in the United States.[10] With expanded numbers of DRGs and/or ICD9s, it will be necessary to have a policing mechanism to prevent widespread "upcoding" to obtain more money for the same services. This system will be used as a basis for

1. Regional electronic billing
2. Capitation payment
3. "Outcomes analysis" with standards of care
4. Quality control throughout the provider/payer network
5. Managed care programs with cost containment responsibility
6. Health care fraud control—will allow database for multiple codes and upcoding
7. Utilization analyses

ELECTRONIC CLAIMS CLEARINGHOUSE

The system outlined in H.R. 5502 "Health Care Cost Containment and Reform Act of 1992"[11] by Representative Fortney "Pete" Stark (D-9-CA) provides for standardized electronic claims, electronic medical records, and electronic claims clearinghouses. Such a system would provide quick and accurate information regarding claims, payments to providers, costs of chronic and catastrophic illnesses and conditions, the quality of care, health care fraud, and other vital cost and administrative information which is necessary to the provision of appropriate medical and health care to qualified recipients.

LONG-TERM CARE

Long-term medical and health care would be limited to *home and hospice care* and would be covered by a combination of the current Medicare system and the Social Security system, with all American citizens and naturalized citizens covered. A strict, but meaningful "means test" would be applied to every recipient with annual auditing. Those persons below the poverty level would have a minimum copayment and deductible limit. A sliding scale would provide that those with gross annual incomes between 100 and 200 percent of the poverty level would pay a reasonable, but minimum premium, copayment, and deductible. Those with gross annual incomes above 200 percent of the poverty level would pay premiums, copayments, and deductibles that would result in complete payment of all long-term care after 300 percent of the poverty level. Irrespective of poverty level status of the recipient of government supported long-term care, a recipient qualified to receive Social Security benefits will be subject to a "first dollar cost" liability of up to 80 percent of such Social Security benefits. After 80 percent of the recipient's Social Security benefits are applied to the costs of his or her long-term care, the remainder of premiums due, copayments and deductibles will apply to other income sources.

The administration, provision of service, and oversight of the long-term care program could be patterned somewhat after the provisions of S. 1446 "Health USA Act of 1991," as introduced to the Committee on Finance by Senator Robert Kerrey (D-NE), in Section 202.[12]

BEHAVIORAL BENEFITS

The treatment of psychological, psychiatric, drug abuse, alcohol abuse, and mental disorders will be limited to 30 days of inpatient care plus 25 days of outpatient care annually for any combination of these illnesses for any person covered under the national plan. There will be a lifetime dollar limit of $100,000 for the treatment or care of any combination of psychological, psychiatric, drug abuse, alcohol abuse, and mental illness for any person covered under the national plan.

WORKERS COMPENSATION

A shortcoming of almost all national plans in the literature is that they do not discuss the treatment of Workers Compensation for the 50 states. Each state operates its own Workers Compensation plan autonomously from any other state plan. All state Workers Compensation plans should be revised so that the responsibility for occupational and non-occupational *medical and health care* previously covered under Workers Compensation is removed from all state Workers Compensation statutes and becomes a part of the general medical and health care provisions of the national health care plan, subject to all the managed care and cost containment provisions of the national health care plan. Since the medical and health care benefits previously covered by the Workers Compensation plans will now be covered under the national health care plan, the premiums charged employers should reflect this "carve out" of benefit responsibility. In those industries where there is an *actuarially determined* unusually high incidence of injuries, that industry must have an actuarially determined

increment added to the 3 percent that the employer pays into the national
health care system.

FUNDING THE NATIONAL PLAN

The primary funding for the national plan will be accomplished through
a National Health Care Fund, administered jointly by the federal and
state governments. The funds for this program will be derived and provided to the National Health Care Fund in the following manner:

1. Employer contribution equal to 3 percent of the gross earnings
   of each wage or salaried employee.
2. Employee contribution of 7 percent of gross earnings, with
   no upper limit.
3. A 1 percent Value Added Tax (VAT) on all consumer durables
   produced in America or imported from foreign nations.
4. For each dollar of foreign aid granted to any foreign government or nation 0.001 percent of such amounts will be provided
   to the National Health Care Fund for national health care in
   America.

Of the combined tax outlined in items 1 and 2 above, one-half of one
percent will go to the federal government for administration of the National Health Care Fund and other administrative activities, and the remainder will remain in the state collecting the taxes. The remaining taxes
will be distributed to the states to implement and maintain their national
health care plans according to a formula to be designed and by a National
Health Care Advisory Board.

The federal government, its agents, or assigns may not withhold, delay,
or obstruct the payment of any national health care funds to states for
the purpose of causing a state to comply with any federal regulation, law,
or executive order.

UNIVERSAL COVERAGE

There are compelling arguments on both sides of the universal coverage
issue. If any kind of universal coverage is adopted, the costs will be
enormous and will require all citizens to both contribute to the national
health care system and contribute to the reduction of the national debt.
It is unlikely that any of the ''piecemeal reforms'' will be able to ac-

complish expanding health care coverage to those who need it most—the underclass—without placing such a heavy burden on employers that they will reduce benefits that they are voluntarily providing now and will terminate the jobs of marginal employees.

The "pay-or-play" should be named "pay-or-pay." Employers *pay* no matter which option they take. That type of system places such penalties on employers and is so inflexible for employers of different sizes and with different employee compositions that employers would have difficulty surviving. Such a system is a cost shifting and responsibility shifting from the federal government to employers. It is the way Congress can look like it is providing some service while employers "pick up the tab." Stuart Butler of The Heritage Foundation challenged the federal government to take a two-pronged course of action: "1. End the link between health care tax breaks and the place of work. 2. Establish a 'Health Care Social Contract.' "

If health care is totally "de-linked" from the workplace and the government makes a social contract with individuals for their own health care, business and industry can go about doing what they should do—making a high quality product at the lowest possible price, while providing a reasonable rate of return to investors.

A national health care plan will stand or fall on the willingness of recipients to pay their fair share of the costs *for their own health care*.

NOTES

1. U.S. House of Representatives, *Long-Term Strategies For Health Care*, Hearings Before the Committee on Ways and Means, House of Representatives, Serial 102–33, 102d Cong., 1st Sess., April 16–17, 23–25, 1991 (Washington, D.C.: U.S. Government Printing Office, 1992) and U.S. House of Representatives, *Oversight Hearing on National Health Care Reform* Serial No. 102–104, 7 May 1992 (Washington, D.C.: U.S. Government Printing Office, 1992).

2. The "pay-or-play" plans discussed at length in chapter 6 were sponsored by Democrats, with the exception of the CHIP plan, S. 2114, sponsored by Senator Bob Packwood (R-OR).

3. President George Bush has supported a system of vouchers to help the poor and underinsured obtain and maintain health care insurance.

4. American Medical Association, "Executive Summary" in testimony before U.S. House of Representatives, *Long-Term Strategies For Health Care, op. cit.*, p. 791.

5. Title 10 (P.L. 99–272), Consolidated Omnibus Budget Reconciliation Act of 1986 (COBRA).

6. Tax Equity and Fiscal Responsibility Act of 1982 (TEFRA).

7. Deficit Reduction Act of 1984 (DEFRA).

8. Title 1 of the Employee Retirement Income Security Act of 1974 (ERISA) as amended by the Retirement Equity Act of 1984 (REA) and by the Tax Reform Act of 1986 (TRA).

9. The National Association of Children's Hospitals and Related Institutions, Inc., before the U.S. House of Representatives, *Long-Term Strategies For Health Care*, *op. cit.*, p. 842.

10. Testimony of Carson Beadle before the U.S. House of Representatives, *Long-Term Strategies For Health Care*, *op. cit.*, pp. 293–307.

11. U.S. House of Representatives, "Health Care Cost Containment and Reform Act of 1992," H.R. 5502, 102d Cong., 2nd Sess. (Washington, D.C.: U.S. Government Printing Office, 1992), Sections 222–223, pp. 89–107.

12. U.S. Senate, "Health USA Act of 1991," S. 1446, 102d Cong., 1st Sess. (Washington, D.C.: U.S. Government Printing Office, 1991), Section 202, pp. 19–25.

13. Testimony before the U.S. House of Representatives, *Long-Term Strategies For Health Care*, *op. cit.*, pp. 697–710.

15

Between Now and 2000 A.D.

Health care scholars believe that the type of health care administrative and delivery network and nature of medical and health benefits that will be offered in the year 2000 and beyond will be radically different from those offered now. Attitudes toward abortion, euthanasia, assisted suicide, resuscitation of underweight babies are just now being formed in the public mind. The ethics of ''pulling the plug'' on medical services for a number of ''terminal'' situations is being debated in the courts and in the privacy of the family unit.

Even with a national health care plan, some of these issues will be magnified as they become more frequent and as they are debated in open forums such as on public radio and television. The emotional and physical pain associated with a terminal cancer patient, a person with Alzheimer's disease, a person with terminal AIDS, an extremely underweight ''crack cocaine'' baby, and a person lying in a persistent, terminal vegetative state are becoming more openly discussed on radio and television programs. How can we not become more empathetic, being drawn into these situations as we are at an increasing rate?

A mandatory national health care plan will guarantee every citizen uniform access to a basic level of health care, irrespective of employment status. By the year 2000, the national health care plan will provide comprehensive benefits for all Americans, including hospital and physician care, dental services and care, long-term care, prescription drugs and durable health care aids, mental health services, and a whole array of preventive care measures. In discussing the universal health care approach like that plan outlined in the previous chapter, Robert Reishauer, Director of the Congressional Budget Office states:

> The plan described here would replace all existing insurance for acute-care services with a new public insurance plan for which all legal residents would be eligible. The benefit package would be actuarially equivalent to the average benefits currently provided under private plans and Medicare. Providers would be paid on the same terms as those now in place under Medicare, financed from broad-based federal and state taxes. Private insurance plans would be prohibited from offering any benefits covered by the public plan, including a prohibition on paying the public plan's copayment requirements (which would be capped). Private plans would, however, be permitted to offer coverage for services not covered by the public plan.[1]

With a national health care identity card, every American citizen will be able to choose his or her own physician or source of medical care. Since the program will be a standard federal program, administered jointly between the federal government and the states, the benefits will be uniform, as will the quality of services and treatment. Will the people be willing to pay for these benefits? John Moynahan, Jr., of the Metropolitan Life Insurance Company believes that the people will be willing to pay. He testifies:

> The first trade-off issue to examine is a practical one: how to pay for universal coverage. One way to finance reform is to reallocate existing resources. Stakeholders were asked if the additional cost of covering 31 million uninsured meant $50 billion less spent on other goods and services—would they favor or oppose such a reallocation? Majorities of most groups favor such a reallocation to cover the uninsured. An alternative to reallocating resources is to raise more revenues. Stakeholders were asked, if it were part of a program in which all made compromises to reach a consensus, how acceptable would higher income taxes be? Higher taxes were *more* acceptable than reallocation of existing funds. More than 65% of all groups found payment of higher income taxes acceptable but corporate executives (at 57%) find higher income taxes less acceptable than other groups. By the way, keep in mind these respondents are sophisticated individuals who likely understand the magnitude of the taxes required.[2]

The national health care plan will take the worry out of transferring from one job to another because all benefits are independent of employment. The unemployed will enjoy the same level of care and health care options as an employed person in the basic plan. Elders will be able to plan for the future with more self-confidence, knowing that health care will be assured in their remaining years.

Probably the greatest benefit of the nationalized system will be the fact that physicians, nurses, and health care specialists will be able to devote their time to taking care of patients rather than filling out endless, complicated forms. The electronic transmission of information will take care of most of the paperwork problem.

Employers will be relieved of their burden to administer health care plans and serve as a proxy for the federal government as a social welfare agency. Since the health care responsibility will be transferred back to the government, where it should have been all along, the employer can devote all of the resources of the firm to making a better product at a cheaper price and give the investors a reasonable rate of return on their investment. This is an economic principle that is simple, yet disregarded by the members of Congress when they try to reduce taxes by shifting their costs and responsibilities to employers. Robert C. Winters of The Business Roundtable agrees that the responsibility shifting has been an impediment to employer-provided health care coverage. He states:

We also oppose federal or state requirements that require employers to provide particular levels or types of health-care benefits. These state-mandated benefits substantially impede the expansion of private insurance coverage of the increasing cost. One study concludes that 16 percent of the firms not offering coverage today would do so in an environment that was free of mandated benefits. The private market can better address the need for coverage if carriers have the latitude to design affordable coverages that their customers want to buy.[3]

The plan proposed in the previous chapter would permit the employer to offer supplemental benefits above and beyond the national health plan coverage if employees were willing to pay for them. The benefits would be tailored to the employees' needs and would be autonomous with regard to any package of benefits offered as a basic plan.

Many of the bills considered by Congress, discussed in chapters 5 through 7 of this book, have very strong health care features. Most of them, however, seek to expand national health care through the employer because this network has already worked well for several million people in the past. These employer-mandate approaches have already proven to weaken the ability of businesses to compete in both domestic and world markets, have created a high level of unemployment, and have penalized the marginal and part-time worker—precisely the target group that most desperately needs basic health care benefits for themselves and their dependents.

Michael Castle, testifying for the National Governors' Association before the U.S. House of Representatives Ways and Means Committee, agrees that Medicaid is not the way to handle long-term care. The plan in chapter 13 provides for a combined program with Medicare and Social Security. The National Governors' Association argued:

> Would it be more appropriate to move long-term care out of the Medicaid program? Because Medicaid is an acute care program with an institutional bias, it may not be the best program to provide long-term care services. In 1989, 43 percent of nursing home care in the United States was paid for by Medicaid. A new program designed to meet both the social and health care needs of the elderly may provide a more appropriate approach to this population. We may even consider a national program for catastrophic and long-term care coverage that could reduce the cost of insurance throughout the health care system.[4]

The plan proposed in the preceding chapter did include such a long-term care strategy which addressed both chronic and catastrophic long-term medical and health care services through a combination of the Medicare network and the Social Security network. Such a combination would consolidate benefits to those who need them most through a single source and would also facilitate the payment of the long-term care costs and any supplemental costs associated with long-term care.

The year 2000 will witness a new health care system, a different political system, and a beginning of a new millennium of people trying to find out ways to live together at the highest possible standard of life with the best possible health. Do we have the right strategies for such a challenge?

The author would be grateful to receive comments or questions regarding any subject contained in this book. Please send comments or queries to the author at:

Webster University
Graduate School
470 East Lockwood Avenue
Saint Louis, MO 63119-3194

NOTES

1. Testimony of Robert Reishauer, Director, Congressional Budget Office, before the U.S. House of Representatives, *Long-Term Strategies For Health Care*, Hearings Before the Committee on Ways and Means, House of Representatives, Serial 102–33, 102d Cong., 1st Sess., April 16–17, 23–25, 1991 (Washington, D.C.: U.S. Government Printing Office, 1992), pp. 408–428.

2. Testimony of John Moynahan, Jr., before the U.S. House of Representatives, *Long-Term Strategies For Health Care*, pp. 796–805.

3. Testimony of Robert C. Winters, The Business Roundtable before the U.S. House of Representatives, *Long-Term Strategies For Health Care, op. cit.*, pp. 431–436.

4. Testimony of Michael N. Castle, Governor of Delaware, National Governors' Association before the U.S. House of Representatives, *Long-Term Strategies For Health Care, op. cit.*, pp. 746–751.

Bibliography

Advisory Commission on Intergovernmental Relations. *MEDICAID Intergovernmental Trends and Options* No. A-119. Washington, D.C.: USACIR, 1992.

Albert, Rory and Neal Schelberg. "Benefit Plans Redefined Under ADEA; Cases and Rulings," *Pension World* (October 1989):45–48.

Altenstetter, Christa. "An End to a Consensus on Health Care in the Federal Republic of Germany?" *Journal of Health Politics, Policy and Law* (Fall 1987):505–536.

Altman, Stuart and Harvey Sapolsky, eds. *Federal Health Programs: Problems and Prospects*. Lexington, Mass.: Lexington Books, 1981.

American College of Physicians. "Access to Health Care," *Annals of Internal Medicine* 112 (May 1990):642–661.

American Hospital Association. *National Health Strategy: A Starting Point for Debate*. Chicago: American Hospital Association, 1991.

Americans with Disabilities Act of 1990, Public Law 101–336 (Title I, S. 933, 101st Cong. and Title II, H.R. 2773, 101st Cong.).

Anderson, Gerard et al. "Capitation Pricing: Adjusting For Prior Utilization And Physician Discretion," *Health Care Financing Review* (Winter 1986):27–34.

Anderson, Kevin. "Small Firms are Getting Squeezed Out," *USA Today*, 13 June 1991, pp. 1B–2B.

Aschkenasy, Janet. "Pepper Panel's Proposed Plan is Criticized: Health Insurers See Pitfalls," *Journal of Commerce and Commercial* (6 March 1990):9A.

"Assessing the Future of Long-Term Care," *Healthspan* (Mar. 1988):6–15.

Bacon, Kenneth H. "Private Drug Abuse Treatment Centers Try to Adjust to Life in the Slow Lane," *The Wall Street Journal*, 23 July 1990, B1, B6.

Barer, Morris and Robert Evans. "Interpreting Canada: Models, Mind-Sets, and Myths," *Health Affairs* (Spring 1992):44–61.

Barer, Morris, Roger Evans, and Roberta Labelle. "Fee Controls As Cost Control: Tales From The Frozen North," *The Milbank Quarterly* 66:1 (1988):1–64.

Barnes, Don. "Health Insurance Bites the Bullet: I," *National Underwriter Life & Health—Financial Services Edition* (5 March 1990):49.

Beadle, Carson E. "The Future Of Employee Benefits: More Mandates Ahead," *Compensation And Benefits Review* (Nov.–Dec. 1988):36–44.

"Behavioral Benefits." *Employee Benefit Plan Review* (Feb. 1990):8–31.

Benjamin, A. E. "Long-term Care And AIDS: Perspectives From Experience With The Elderly," *The Milbank Quarterly* 66:3 (1988):415–443.

Blank, Robert H. *Rationing Medicine.* New York: Columbia University Press, 1988.

Blendon, Robert. "Three Systems: A Comparative Survey," *Health Management Quarterly* (First Quarter, 1989):2–10.

Boekhoff, Jay and Robert Dobson. "The Long Term Care Insurance Challenge," *Emphasis* (Oct. 1987):6–8.

Borzi, Paul C. "Summary of Health Insurance Coverage Act of 1985 (Title X of The Consolidated Omnibus Budget Reconciliation Act of 1985, P.L. 99–272), as Amended by Section 1895(d) of The Tax Reform Act of 1986" U.S. House of Representatives, Committee on Labor-Management Relations.

Boyd, Bruce and Alyse Hoyos. "Long Term Care—A Retirement Planning," *Benefits Quarterly* vol. 3 (1987):1–9.

Brandt, Larry and Pam Steiner-Grossman, eds. *Treating IBD; A Patient's Guide to the Medical and Surgical Management of Inflammatory Bowel Disease.* New York: Raven Press, 1989.

Brasfield, James. "Health Planning Reform: A Proposal for the Eighties," *Journal of Health Politics, Policy and Law* (Winter 1982):718–738.

Bresch, Jack and Frederick Krebs. "Compulsory Employee Benefits: Pro And Con," *Association Management* (April 1989):86–91.

Brigham, Karen. "Finding the Best Prescription for the Nation's Health-Care Woes," *Congressional Action (Special Report)* U. S. Chamber of Commerce (June 26 1989):1–4.

"Broad Change Sought For Health System." *Employee Benefit Plan Review* (Mar. 1990):31–32.

Brostoff, Steven. "Medigap Rate Legislation Introduced In House," *National Underwriter* (5 March 1990):4, 53.

Brown, Lawrence D. "Introduction To A Decade Of Transition," *Journal Of Health Politics, Policy And Law* 16 (1986):569–570.

Brown, Richard. "Principles for a National Health Program: A Framework for Analysis and Development," *The Milbank Quarterly* 4 (1988):573–617.

Bruzzese, Anita. "Companies Cut Retiree Benefits," *Employee Benefit News* Vol. 1 (Apr. 1987):1, 36.

Bryant, Bertha. "Issues on the Distribution of Health Care: Some Lessons from Canada," *Public Health Reports* (September–October 1981):442–447.

Buchanan, Allen. "Competition, Charity, and the Right to Health Care" in Attig, Thomas, et al., ed., *The Restraint of Liberty.* Bowling Green, Ohio: Bowling Green State University, 1985:129–143.

Buchi, Kenneth and Bruce Landesman. "Health Care in a National Health Program: A Fundamental Right" in Huefner, Robert and Margaret Battin, eds., *Changing to National Health Care: Ethical and Policy Issues.* Salt Lake City, Utah: University of Utah Press, 1992, pp. 191–208.

Burgdorf, Robert, Jr. "Equal Access to Public Accommodations," *The Milbank Quarterly* Supp. 1/2, 69 (1991):183–213.

Bush, Gerald W. et al. "Prefunding of Postretirement Health Care Services," *Compensation & Benefits Management* 3 (Spring 1987):85–92.

Butler, Patricia and Robert Schlenker. "Case-mix Reimbursement For Nursing Homes: Objectives And Achievements," *The Milbank Quarterly*, 67:1 (1989):103–136.

Butler, Stuart. "Using Tax Credits to Create an Affordable National Health System," *The Heritage Foundation Backgrounder* No. 777 (20 July 1990).

Butler, Stuart and Edmund Haislmaier. *A National Health System for America*. Washington, D.C.: The Heritage Foundation, 1989.

Caldwell, B. "Health Lawyers Probe the Cost and Quality Nexus," *Employee Benefit Plan Review* (Aug. 1989):30–31.

Callahan, David. *Setting Limits: Medical Goals In An Aging Society*. New York: Touchstone/Simon & Schuster, 1987.

Campion, Frank. *The AMA and U.S. Health Policy: Since 1940*. Chicago: Chicago Review Press, 1984.

Cantor, Joel. "Expanding Health Insurance Coverage: Who Will Pay?" *Journal of Health Politics, Policy and Law* (Winter 1990):755–778.

Caplan, A. L. "A New Dilemma: Quality, Ethics and Expensive Medical Technologies," *The New York Medical Quarterly* 6 (1986):23–27.

Carlsen, Melody A. "Growing Uncertainties—Mandated Benefits And Long Term Care," *CEBS Census of Certified Benefit Specialists* (May 1988).

"Changes in Health Care Costs and Utilization Associated With Mental Health Treatment." *Medical Benefits* (31 Oct. 1987):4.

Chirikos, Thomas. "The Economics of Employment" in West, Jane, ed., *The Americans with Disabilities Act: From Policy to Practice*. New York: Milbank Memorial Fund, 1991:150–179.

Churchill, L. R. *Rationing Health Care In America: Perceptions And Principles Of Justice*. Notre Dame: University of Notre Dame Press, 1987.

Clay, Joan. "The Child Care Issue: Benefits Required By A Changing Workforce," *Employee Benefits Journal* (Sept. 1989):32–34.

Cleverley, William O. *Essentials Of Health Care Finance* 2nd ed. Rockville: Aspen Publishers, 1986.

Clift, Eleanor and Mary Hager. "A Victory for the Haves? Lawmakers Trim Back Catastrophic Health Care," *Newsweek* (16 Oct. 1989):38.

Cohen, Marc, Nanda Kumar, and Stanley Wallack. "Who Buys Long-Term Care Insurance?" *Health Affairs* (Spring 1992):208–223.

"Commission Proposes Benefits Mandate." *Employee Benefit Plan Review* (May 1990):52–54.

"Congress Considers Family Leaves." *Business Insurance* (2 Apr. 1990):6.

Congressional Budget Office. *Selected Options for Expanding Health Insurance Coverage*. Washington, D.C.: U.S. Government Printing Office, 1991, p. xii.

Congressional Budget Office. "Trends in Health Expenditures by Medicare and the Nation," Washington, D.C.: U.S. Government Printing Office, 1991.

Congressional Budget Office. *Rising Health Care Costs: Causes, Implications, and Strategies*. Washington, D.C.: CBO, 1991.

"Consolidated Omnibus Budget Reconciliation Act of 1985 (Public Law 99–272)." *Health Care Financing Review* (Spring 1987):95–115.

"Continuation Of Coverage Lawsuits Begin." *Employee Benefit Plan Review* (Jan. 1990):73–75.

"Cost, Utilization Trends In Psych, Drug Abuse." *Employee Benefit Plan Review* (Feb. 1990):12–13.

"The Crisis in Health Insurance." *Consumer Reports* (Aug. 1990):533–549.

Curtis, Thomas and Donald Westerfield. *Congressional Intent*. New York: Praeger, 1992.

Daley, Susan J. "The Meaning Of Mandated Health Benefits," *Corporate Health* (July/Aug. 1988):12–15.

Daniels, Norman. "Is the Oregon Rationing Plan Fair?" *Journal of the American Medical Association* 265 (1991):232–235.

Danzon, Patricia. "Hidden Overhead Costs: Is Canada's System Less Expensive?" *Health Affairs* (Spring 1992):21–43.

David, H. P. et al., eds. *Born Unwanted: Developmental Effects Of Denied Abortion*. New York: Springer, 1988.

Davis, Karen and Cathy Schoen. *Health and the War on Poverty: A Ten-Year Appraisal*. Washington, D.C.: The Brookings Institution, 1978.

"Deflating Health Costs Through Strategic Plan Design." *Employee Benefit Plan Review* (Dec. 1989):14–16.

Delaney, Meg. "KSOPs: A Marriage of Convenience," *Employee Benefits* 12 (Dec. 1987):24–26.

Delaney, Meg. "Who Will Pay For Retiree Health Care?" *Personnel Journal* 66 (Mar. 1987):82–91.

Diblasie, D. "Managed Care Eases Pain Of Transplant Costs," *Business Insurance* (19 Feb. 1990):3–4, 6.

Dobson, Allen and Elizabeth Hoy. "Hospital PPS Profits: Past And Prospective," *Health Affairs* (Spring 1988):126–129.

Donahue, Richard J. "AIDS Cost Could Lead to National Health Insurance Plan," *National Underwriter* (9 Nov. 1987):6, 46.

Dopkeen, Jonathan C. "Post-Retirement Benefits: A Bottomless Liability?" *Business And Health* 4 (June 1987):9–14.

Dosier, L. and L. Hamilton. "Social Responsibility and Your Employer," *Personnel Administrator* (Apr. 1989):88, 90, 92, 95.

Doty, Pamela, Korbin Liu, and Joshua Wiener. "An Overview Of Long-Term Care," *Health Care Financing Review* (Spring 1985):69–78.

Droste, Therese. "Will Employers Accept a National Health Plan?" *Hospitals* (20 May 1989):81.

Duff, David and Amy Taylor. "Postretirement Welfare Benefits: A New Look at Old Commitments," *Compensation and Benefits Review* (Sept.–Oct. 1989):17–28.

Dwyer, Paula. "At This Medical Lab, Only The Bills Were Real," *Business Week* (16 Oct. 1989):38.

Eddy, David. "Rationing by Patient Choice," *Journal of the American Medical Association* 265 (1991):105–108.

Edwards, Jennifer, et al. "Small Business and the National Health Care Reform Debate," *Health Affairs* (Spring 1992):164–173.

"Employers Would Cut Wages, Benefits, If Minimum Health Care Bill Becomes Law." *Benefits Today* (6 Nov. 1987):384.

Enthoven, Alain. "Managed Competition: An Agenda for Action," *Health Affairs* (Summer 1988):25–47.

Enthoven, Alain and Richard Kronick. "A Consumer-Choice Health Plan for the 1990s," [part 1] *The New England Journal of Medicine* 320 (January 1989):29–37.

Enthoven, Alain and Richard Kronick. "A Consumer-Choice Health Plan for the 1990s," [part 2] *The New England Journal of Medicine* 320 (January 1989):94–101.

Evans, Robert. *Strained Mercy: The Economics of Canadian Health Care.* Toronto: Butterworth, 1984.

Evans, Robert, et al. "Controlling Health Expenditures—The Canadian Reality," *New England Journal of Medicine* (2 March 1989):571–577.

Farrell, Christopher. "The Age Wave—And How To Ride It," *Business Week* (16 Oct. 1989):112, 116.

Fein, Rashi. "Prescription for Change," *Modern Maturity* (August–September 1992):22–35.

Feldblum, Chai. "Employment Protections," *The Milbank Quarterly* Supp. 1/2, 69 (1991):81–110.

Feldstein, Paul. *The Politics of Health Legislation: An Economic Perspective.* Ann Arbor, Michigan: Health Administration Press, 1988.

Feldstein, Paul. "Why the United States Has Not Had National Health Insurance" in Huefner, Robert and Margaret Battin, eds., *Changing to National Health Care: Ethical and Policy Issues.* Salt Lake City, Utah: University of Utah Press, 1992:51–71.

Feldstein, Paul, T. M. Wickizer, and J. R. Wheeler. "The Effect of Utilization Review Programs on Health Care Use and Expenditures," *The New England Journal Of Medicine* (19 May 1988):1310–1314.

Feuer, Dale. "Workplace Issues: Testing, Training and Policy," *Training* 24 (Oct. 1987):66–72.

Field, Marilyn and Bradford Gray. "Should We Regulate 'Utilization Management?'," *Health Affairs* (Winter 1989):103–112.

Finkel, Madelon and Hirsch Ruchlin. *Retiree Health Care: A Ticking Time Bomb.* Brookfield, Wisconsin: International Foundation of Employee Benefit Plans, 1988.

Fisher, M. J. "Health Cover Mandate Proposed," *National Underwriter* (1 June 1987):3, 95.

Foley, Jill. "Uninsured in the United States: The Nonelderly Population Without Health Insurance," Employee Benefit Research Institute (EBRI), Special Report SR-10 (April 1991).

Fossett, J. W., J. A. Peterson, and M. C. Ring. "Public Sector Primary Care And Medicaid: Trading Accessibility For Mainstreaming," *Journal Of Health Politics, Policy And Law* 14 (Fall 1989):309–325.

Francis, John. "Lessons from Abroad in Assessing National Health Care Systems: Ethics and Decision Making" in Huefner, Robert and Margaret Battin, eds., *Changing to National Health Care: Ethical and Policy Issues.* Salt Lake City, Utah: University of Utah Press, 1992:79–106.

Frank, R. G. "Regulatory Policy And Information Deficiencies In The Market For Mental Health Services," *Journal Of Health Politics, Policy and Law* 14 (Fall 1989):477–501.

Frieden, J. "Cost Containment Strategies for Workers' Compensation," *Business and Health* (Oct. 1989):48–50, 52–54.

Frieden, J. "Getting Your Flexible Benefits Program Under Way," *Business and Health* (Oct. 1989):44, 46–47.

"Future Of Flexible Plans Examined." *Employee Benefit Plan Review* (Aug. 1989):47–48.

Gabel, Jon et al. "The Changing World Of Group Health Insurance," *Health Affairs* (Summer 1988):48–65.

Gabel, Jon et al. "Employer-Sponsored Health Insurance in America," *Health Affairs* (Summer 1989):116–128.

Galen, M. "Are Companies Cutting Too Close To The Bone?" *Business Week* (30 Oct. 1989):141, 144.

Garland, Susan B. "America's Child-Care Crisis: The First Tiny Steps Toward Solutions," *Business Week* (10 July 1989):64–68.

Garland, Susan, ed. "The Torpedo That Slammed Into Catastrophic Health Care," *Business Week* (23 Oct. 1989):70.

Garland, Susan and Tim Smart. "Hospitals: Damned If They Merge, Damned If They Don't," *Business Week* (6 Nov. 1989):48–50.

Geisel, Jerry. "Firms Assess Value Of Cost Control," *Business Insurance* (5 Feb. 1990):5, 23–25.

Geisel, Jerry. "Firms Fret About Retiree Health Care Liabilities," *Business Insurance* (28 Dec. 1987):19.

Geisel, Jerry. "National Health Insurance Faulted: 94% of Executives Polled Oppose Idea," *Business Insurance* (2 April 1990):54.

Geisel, Jerry. "Retiree Health Rules To Cut Profits: Study," *Business Insurance* (23 Nov. 1987):27–28.

Ginsburg, Paul. "Physician Payment Policy In The 101st Congress," *Health Affairs* (Spring 1989):5–20.

"Giving Employees Time, Flexibility." *Employee Benefit Plan Review* (May 1990):16–18.

Glaser, William. "Lessons from Germany: Some Reflections Occasioned by Schulenberg's Report," *Journal of Health Politics, Policy and Law* (Summer 1983):352–365.

Godt, Paul. "Confrontation, Consent and Corporatism: State Strategies and the Medical Profession in France, Great Britain, and West Germany," *Journal of Health Politics, Policy and Law* 16 (Fall 1987):459–480.

Gold, Marsha and Dennis Hodges. "Health Maintenance Organizations In 1988," *Health Affairs* (Winter 1989):125–138.

Goldberger, Susan. "The Politics of Universal Access: The Massachusetts Health Security Act of 1988," *Journal of Health Politics, Policy and Law* (Winter 1990):857–885.

Goldfield, Norbert and Seth Goldsmith, eds. *Alternative Delivery Systems*. Rockville, Maryland: Aspen Publishers, 1987.

Goldsmith, Jeff. "A Radical Prescription for Hospitals," *Harvard Business Review* (May–June 1989):104–110.

Gornick, Marian et al. "Twenty Years of Medicare and Medicaid: Covered Populations, Use of Benefits, and Program Expenditures," *Health Care Financing Review*

1985 Annual Supplement. Washington, D.C.: Health Care Financing Administration, 1985.

Gostin, Lawrence. "Public Health Powers: The Imminence of Radical Change," *The Milbank Quarterly* Supp. 1/2, 69 (1991):268–290.

Graddy, Elizabeth. "Interest Groups or the Public Interest—Why Do We Regulate Health Occupations?" *Journal of Health Politics, Policy and Law* (Spring 1991):25–49.

Graskamp, Ernest. "Long Term Incentives for Management, Part 2: Stock Price Appreciation Grants," *Compensation and Benefits Review* (Sept.–Oct. 1989):29–43.

Gravelle, George and Jay Taylor. "Financing Long Term Care for the Elderly," *National Tax Journal* (Sept. 1989):219–232.

Greenwald, Judy. "Employer Coalitions Offer Purchasing Clout," *Business Insurance* (19 Feb. 1990):3–4, 6.

Guralnik, Jack, Machiko Yanagishita, and Edward L. Schneider. "Projecting The Older Population Of The United States: Lessons From The Past And Prospects For The Future," *The Milbank Quarterly* 66:2 (1988):283–308.

Hadley, Jack, Earl Steinberg, and Judith Feder. "Comparison of Uninsured and Privately Insured Hospital Patients: Condition on Admission, Resource Use, and Outcome," *Journal of the American Medical Association* 265 (16 January 1991):374–379.

Haislmaier, Edmund. "Making Long-Term Health Care More Affordable," *The Heritage Foundation Backgrounder* No. 755 (23 February 1990).

Ham, Christopher. *Health Policy in Britain: The Politics and Organization of the National Health Service*. London: Macmillan, 1985.

Hanley, M. P. "Disability Insurance Protects Key Executives and Company," *Small Business Reports* (Oct. 1989):37–40.

Harrigan, Brian and Nancy Jones. "The Cost Impact of AIDS on Employee Benefits Programs," *Compensation & Benefits Management* Vol. 3 (Winter 1987):27–29.

"Hay Report Shows Trends Toward Cost Shifting in Medical Plans, Capital Accumulation Pension Plans." *Employee Benefit Plan Review* (Aug. 1989):18–19.

"Health Care Coverage by Age, Sex, Race, and Family Income: United States, 1986." *Medical Benefits* (31 Oct. 1987):3–4.

Health Insurance Association of America. *Conventional Health Plans: A Decade Later*. Washington, D.C.: HIAA, Nov. 1988.

Health Insurance Association of America. *Health Care Financing for all Americans*. Washington, D.C.: HIAA, 1991.

Health Policy Agenda Steering Committee. "Health Policy Agenda for the American People," *Journal of the American Medical Association* 257 (1987):1199–1210.

Hearne, Paul. "Employment Strategies for People with Disabilities: A Prescription for Change," *The Milbank Quarterly* Supp. 1/2, 69 (1991):111–128.

Helitzer, J. B. "Coordination-of-Benefits Rules vs. COBRA; State Developments in Employee Benefits," *Benefits Law Journal* (Autumn 1989):401–412.

Heller, R. D. "Cafeteria Benefits Plans: A Simpler Approach; Outlook On Compensation And Benefits," *Personnel* (June 1988):30, 34–35.

Hendershot, Gerry. "Health Status And Medical Care Utilization," *Health Affairs* (Spring 1988):114–121.

Hernon, Peter. "Critically Ill Infants Pose Sad Dilemma: Some Question Life at any Cost," *Saint Louis Post Dispatch* (14 June 1992), pp. 1, 6.

Hiatt, Howard. *America's Health in the Balance: Choice or Chance?* New York: Harper & Row, 1987.

Hickey, John and Kwasha Lipton. "FASB Standards: Ideas for Coping With Bleak Implications of New Accounting," *Benefits* (Feb. 1990):9–12, 28–30.

Hill, Fred P. "What Massachusetts Means To Employers," *Health Cost Management* (May/June 1988):17–21.

Himmelstein, David et al. "A National Health Program for the United States," *New England Journal of Medicine* 320 (January 1989):102–108.

Holahan, John and Sheila Zedlewski. "Insuring Low-Income Americans Through Medicaid Expansion," Urban Institute Working Paper No. 3836–02 (December 1989).

Holahan, John and Stephen Zuckerman. "Medicare Mandatory Assignment: An Unnecessary Risk?" *Health Affairs* (Spring 1989):65–80.

Holzman, David. "Endless Care With Costs To Match," *Insight* (Dec.–Jan. 1987):44–46.

Hornor, Edith, ed. *Almanac of the 50 States: Basic Data Profiles with Comparative Tables.* Washington, D.C.: Information Publications, 1992.

Howard, Lisa S. "Health Providers Blamed For Ranks Of Uninsureds," *National Underwriter* (10 Oct. 1988):5–6.

Huefner, Robert and Margaret Battin, eds. *Changing to National Health Care: Ethical and Policy Issues.* Salt Lake City, Utah: University of Utah Press, 1992.

Humber, James and Robert Almeder, eds. *Biomedical Ethics and the Law.* New York: Plenum Press, 1976.

Institute of Medicine. *The Future of Public Health.* Washington, D.C.: National Academy Press, 1988.

Insurance Information Institute. *Workers' Compensation Insurance: Protecting America's Workers.* New York: Insurance Information Institute, 1981.

Jencks, Stephen and George Schieber. "Containing U.S. Health Care Costs: What Bullet to Bite?" *Health Care Financing Review: 1991 Annual Supplement.* Baltimore, MD: Health Care Financing Administration, 1992.

Jensen, Gail, Michael Morrisey, and John Marcus. "Cost Sharing And The Changing Pattern Of Employer-Sponsored Health Benefits," *The Milbank Quarterly* 65:4 (1987):521–550.

Johns, Lucy and Gerald Adler. "Evaluation Of Recent Changes In Medicaid," *Health Affairs* (Spring 1989):171–181.

Joint Economic Committee. "Health Care Briefing Paper" presented in U.S. House of Representatives. *Oversight Hearing on National Health Care Reform* Serial No. 102–104 (7 May 1992). Washington, D.C.: U.S. Government Printing Office, 1992, pp. 4–33.

Jones, Nancy. "Essential Requirements of the Act: A Short History and Overview," *The Milbank Quarterly* Supp. 1/2, 69 (1991):25–54.

Jones, Woodrow and Mitchell Rice, eds. *Health Care Issues in Black America: Policies, Problems, and Prospects.* New York: Greenwood Press, 1987.

Joseph, E. C. "The Shape of the Future—Visions for Employee Benefits," *Employee Benefits Digest* 27 (Jan. 1990):1, 4–7, 10.

Kantrowitz, Barbara et al. "Now, Parents on Trial (Cocaine Babies: The Littlest Victims)," *Newsweek* (2 Oct. 1989):54–55.

Kantrowitz, Barbara et al. "The Crack Children," *Newsweek* (12 Feb. 1990):62–63.

Katz, David M. "Politicians Clash On Health Benefits Mandates," *National Underwriter* (16 May 1988):52.

Kilner, John. *Who Lives? Who Dies? Ethical Criteria in Patient Selection*. New Haven, Connecticut: Yale University Press, 1990.

Koff, Theodore. *New Approaches to Health Care for an Aging Population: Developing a Continuum of Chronic Care Services*. San Francisco: Jossey-Bass Publishers, 1988.

Koretz, Gene. "Economic Trends," *Business Week* (4 December 1989):24.

Koretz, Gene. "Child Care: A Key To Cutting Welfare Rolls?" *Business Week* (25 Dec. 1989):34.

Kronick, Richard. "The Slippery Slope of Health Care Finance: Business Interests and Hospital Reimbursement in Massachusetts," *Journal of Health Politics, Policy and Law* (Winter 1990):887–913.

Krueger, Judy K. "Mandated Health Care And Small Business: Does Anyone Win?" *Mid America Insurance* (July 1988):26–30.

Kutz, Karen S. "Chandler Bill Supports Retiree Insurance," *Pension World* Vol. 23 (August 1987):8–9.

Landes, Jennifer. "Group Health Cost Per Employee Hit High In '89," *Life & Health/ Financial Services* (19 Feb. 1990):3, 12–13.

Lapidus, M. "The Proposed Regulations Under Internal Revenue Code Section 89 And 125: An Overview," *Tax Management Compensation Planning Journal* (May 1989):95–105.

LaPlante, Mitchell. "The Demographics of Disability," *The Milbank Quarterly* Supp. 1/2, 69 (1991):55–77.

Laudicina, Susan. "State Health Risk Pools: Insuring The 'Uninsurable'," *Health Affairs* (Fall 1988):97–104.

Lautzenheiser, Barbara. "Socialized Insurance: The Rising Tide," *Best's Review: Life & Health Insurance Edition* (Jan. 1989):22–24, 104.

Laverty, C. "A Well-Kept Secret: Insurers Ignoring Savings Of Home Health Care," *Business Insurance* (12 Feb. 1990):19.

"Legal Climate Clears Over Retiree Health Benefits." *Employee Benefit Plan Review* Vol. 41 (June 1987):8–10.

Levin, Arthur, ed. *Regulating Health Care: The Struggle for Control*. New York: The Academy of Political Science, 1980.

Levit, Katharine and Cathy Cowan. "Burden of Health Care Costs: Business, Households, and Government," *Health Care Financing Review* 12(2):127–137. HCFA Pub. No. 03316. Washington, D.C.: HCFA, 1990.

Levit, Katharine and Cathy Cowan. "Business, Households, and Governments: Health Care Costs, 1990," *Health Care Financing Review* (Winter 1991):83–102.

Levit, Katharine, Mark Freeland, and Daniel Waldo. "Health Spending and Ability to Pay: Business, Individuals, and Government," *Health Care Financing Review* 10(3):1–11 HFCA Pub. No. 03280. Washington, D.C.: HCFA, 1989.

Levit, Katharine, Helen Lazenby, Cathy Cowan, Suzanne Letsch. "National Health Expenditures, 1990," *Health Care Financing Review* 13(1):29–54 HCFA Pub. No. 03321. Washington, D.C.: HCFA, 1991.

Light, Donald, et al. "Social Medicine vs. Professional Dominance: The German Experience," *American Journal of Public Health* (January 1986):78–83.

Light, Larry. "The Power Of The Pension Funds," *Business Week* (6 Nov. 1989):154–158.

Lister, John. "The Politics of Medicine in Britain and the United States," *New England Journal of Medicine* (17 July 1986):168–173.

Lister, John. "Proposals for Reform of the British National Health Service," *New England Journal of Medicine* (30 March 1989):877–880.

Litman, Theodor and Leonard Robins. *Health Politics and Policy*, 2nd ed. New York: Delmar Publishers, 1991, p. 80.

Long, Stephen and Jack Rogers. "The Effects of Being Uninsured on Health Care Service Use Estimates from the Survey of Income and Program Participation," *Survey of Income and Program Participation (SIPP) Working Paper No. 9012*. Washington, D.C.: Bureau of the Census, 1990.

Lubeck, Deborah and Edward Yelin. "A Question Of Value: Measuring The Impact Of Chronic Disease," *The Milbank Quarterly* 66:3 (1988):444–464.

Luft, Harold and Robert Miller. "Patient Selection In A Competitive Health System," *Health Affairs* (Summer 1988):97–119.

McConnell, Campbell and Stanley Brue. *Economics* 11th ed. Saint Louis: McGraw-Hill, 1990.

McDonnell, Patricia et al. "Self-Insured Health Plans," *Health Care Financing Review* (Winter 1986):1–14.

McMenamin, Peter. "Medicare Part B Carrier Approved Charges in 1988," *Health Affairs* (Fall 1989):205–211.

Mechanic, David. *Future Issues in Health Care: Social Policy and the Rationing of Medical Services*. New York: The Free Press, 1979.

Mechanic, David. "Consumer Choice Among Health Insurance Options," *Health Affairs* (Spring 1989):138–148.

"Medical Necessity: Health Care's Third Revolution?" *Employee Benefit Plan Review* (Aug. 1989):32, 34.

Meilicke, Carl and Janet Storch, eds. *Perspectives on Canadian Health and Social Services Policy: History and Emerging Trends*. Ann Arbor, Michigan: Health Administration Press, 1980.

Meyer, Jack, ed. *Market Reforms in Health Care: Current Issues, New Directions, Strategic Decisions*. Washington, D.C.: American Enterprise Institute for Public Policy Research, 1983.

Miccolis, Jerry. "Workers' Compensation—The State of the System," *Emphasis* (1991/1992):15–17.

Miller, Anetta and Mary Hager. "The Elderly Duke It Out," *Newsweek* (11 Sept. 1989):42–43.

Minc, G. J. "Providing A Section 129 Dependent Care Assistance Program Through A Section 125 Cafeteria Plan," *Taxes* (May 1988):361–367.

"Minimum Health Benefits Bill Said Jeopardy to Low-Wage Jobs." *Daily Labor Report* (5 Nov. 1987):A10–A12.

Monheit, Alan and Pamela Short. "Mandating Health Coverage For Working Americans," *Health Affairs* (Winter 1989):22–38.

Mor, Vincent, John Piette, and John Fleishman. "Community-Based Case Management For Persons With AIDS," *Health Affairs* (Winter 1989):139–153.

Morrisey, Michael A. and Gail A. Jensen. "Regional Variation In Health Insurance Coverage," *Health Affairs* (Fall 1989):91–103.

Moyer, Eugene. "A Revised Look At The Number Of Uninsured Americans," *Health Affairs* (Summer 1989):102–110.

Mullen, P. "Mandated Benefits May Be Out Of Reach For Small Firms," *HealthWeek* (27 Dec. 1989):16.

Mullenholz, John. "Repeal Of Section 89—What Now?" *F & P Equipment Dealer* (Dec. 1989):22–25.

Munoz, Eric et al. "Race, DRGs, And The Consumption Of Hospital Resources," *Health Affairs* (Spring 1989):182–190.

Nathans, Leah. "The New Breed Of Pensions That May Leave Retirees Poorer," *Business Week* (6 Nov. 1989):164–167.

National Commission on State Workmen's Compensation Laws. *The Report of the National Commission on State Workmen's Compensation Laws.* Washington, D.C.: U.S. Government Printing Office, 1972.

"National Health Expenditures, 1986–2000." *Health Care Financing Review* (Summer 1987):1–36.

"National Health Expenditures, 1986–2000." *Medical Benefits* (Oct. 1987):1–3.

"Nearly One-Fifth of Plan's Rates Due to State-Mandated Medical Coverage." *Benefits Today* (18 Nov. 1988):378.

Nelson, P. G. "Post-Retirement Benefits: The Tip of a Financial Iceberg." *Management Accounting* (Jan. 1987):52–55.

"New Cafeteria Plan Rules Under IRS Section 125." *BeneNet Spotlight* No. 89–3 (10 Mar. 1989):1–6.

Newhouse, J. P. "Rate Adjusters For Medicare Under Capitation," *Health Care Financing Review* (Supp. 1986):45–55.

Newman, William, James Logan, and Harvey Hegarty. *Strategy: A Multi-Level, Integrative Approach.* Cincinnati: South-Western Publishing Co., 1989, p. 523.

Nickel, James. *Making Sense of Human Rights.* Berkley, California: University of California Press, 1987.

Nirtaut, Dennis J. "Positive Selection: Legislation, Pricing Give HMOs Competitive Edge," *Business Insurance* (11 Sept. 1990):39.

"Now that Section 89 is History, Get Re-Acquainted With Some Old Friends: Sections 79 and 105(h)," *Benefits* (Feb. 1990):7–8, 30.

Nyman, J. A. and C. R. Geyer. "Promoting The Quality Of Life In Nursing Homes: Can Regulation Succeed?" *Journal Of Health Politics, Policy And Law* 14 (Winter 1989):797–816.

Ostuw, Richard. "How Can Employers Cope With Soaring Retiree Health Costs?" *Pension World* Vol. 23 (Mar. 1987):53–55.

Pavuk, A. "Access To Care: The AHA's Position On Mandated Employee Health Benefits," *American Hospital Association, Trustee* (Feb. 1990):12–13, 26.

Pepper Commission—U.S. Bipartisan Commission on Comprehensive Health Care. *A Call For Action.* Washington, D.C.: U.S. Government Printing Office, 1990.

Peppers, Lawrence and David Balls. *Managerial Economics: Theory and Applications for Decision Making.* Englewood Cliffs: Prentice-Hall, 1987.

Perlmutter, C. "15 Reasons To Say 'No' To Hysterectomy," *Prevention* (June 1989):51–59.

Polich, Cynthia, et al. "All For One . . . Government Must Encourage Firms to Offer Retiree Health Plans," *Business Insurance* Vol 21 (24 Aug. 1987):19–20.

Potter, E. E. "Congressionally Mandated Employee Benefits: How Do They Affect

Human Resources And Employment Policy?'' *Compensation & Benefits Management* (Summer 1988):269–272.

Pozgar, George. *Legal Aspects of Health Care Administration* 4th ed. Rockville, Maryland: Aspen Publishers, 1990.

Priester, Reinhard. "A Values Framework for Health System Reform," *Health Affairs* (Spring 1992):84–107.

"Public And Private Issues In Financing Health Care For Children." *ERBI Issue Brief* (June 1989):1–15.

"Public Favors Mandatory Coverage Sponsored by Employers, EBRI Finds." *Benefits Today* (22 Sept. 1989):310–311.

"Rand Study Identifies Unnecessary Procedures." *Employee Benefit Plan Review* (Aug. 1989):35.

Rappaport, Anna and Robert Kalman. "Vesting Issues in Retiree Medical Plans," *Business And Health* 4 (June 1987):24, 26–28.

Reagan, M. "Health Care Rationing: A Problem In Ethics And Policy (Review Essay)," *Journal of Health Politics, Policy And Law* 14 (Fall 1989):627–633.

"Reason Momentarily Overcomes Congress in Late-Night Repeal of IRC Sec. 89 Rules." *Employee Benefit Plan Review* (Dec. 1989):36–37.

Rice, Thomas, Jon Gabel, and Gregory de Lissovoy. "PPOs: The Employer Perspective," *Journal Of Health Politics, Policy And Law* 14:2 (Summer 1989):367–382.

Rocap, D. E. "Golden Parachute Proposed Regs. Clarify Many Issues," *Journal of Taxation* (Oct. 1989):204–210.

Roemer, Milton. *National Health Systems of the World*. New York: Oxford University Press, 1991.

Roemer, Ruth and George McKay. *Legal Aspects of Health Policy: Issues and Trends* Westport, Connecticut: Greenwood Press, 1980.

Rooney, J. Patrick. "Mandating Health Care Would Eliminate Jobs," *Nation's Business* (May 1988):4.

Rosenbloom, J. S. *The Handbook of Employee Benefits: Design, Funding, and Administration* 2nd ed. Homewood: Dow Jones-Irwin, 1988.

Rowland, Diane. "Measuring the Elderly's Need for Home Care," *Health Affairs* (Winter 1989):39–51.

Ryan, K. M. "A System Out of Balance," *Best's Review* (July 1989):54–56, 95.

Sakala, Carol. "The Development of National Medical Care Programs in the United Kingdom and Canada: Applicability to Current Conditions in the United States," *Journal of Health Politics, Policy and Law* (Winter 1990):709–753.

Schaffer, Daniel. "Tax Incentives," *The Milbank Quarterly* Supp. 1/2, 69 (1991):293–312.

Schell, W. M. "Taxes: Cafeteria Plans," *Management Accounting* (May 1989):11.

Schenck, Benjamin R. "Compulsory Health Cover: Pros And Cons," *National Underwriter* (1 Aug. 1988):28–38.

Schmitz, Anthony. "Taking Cover in Ohio, New York, and Oregon," *In Health* (January/February 1991):41.

Schnachner, Mary. "Monsanto To Launch Flex Plan On Jan. 1," *Business Insurance* (27 Nov. 1989):6–7.

Schnachner, Mary. "Parental Leave Endorsed," *Business Insurance* (16 Mar. 1990):2, 38.

Schwartz, William and Henry Aaron. "Rationing Hospital Care: Lessons from Britain," *New England Journal of Medicine* (5 January 1984):52–56.

Seligmann, Jean et al. "Medical Professionals Are Demanding More Effective AIDS Protection For Themselves," *Newsweek* (20 Nov. 1989):82–83.

Shah, B. "An Overview of Pharmaceutical Cost-Containment Practices in the Managed Care Sector," *Drug Benefits Trends* (Feb./Mar. 1989):16–22.

Sheils, John, Gary Young, and Robert Rubin. "O Canada: Do We Expect Too Much from its Health System?" *Health Affairs* (Spring 1992):7–20.

Sheingold, Steven. "The First Three Years Of PPS: Impact On Medicare Costs," *Health Affairs* (Fall 1989):191–204.

Shortell, Stephen. "A Model for State Health Care Reform," *Health Affairs* (Spring 1992):108–127.

Sloan, Frank, Michael Morrisey, and Joseph Valvona. "Effects On the Medicare Prospective Payment System On Hospital Cost Containment: An Early Appraisal," *The Milbank Quarterly* 66:2 (1988):191–220.

"Small Business Pooling Arrangements Called Promising Health Coverage Alternative." *Daily Labor Report* (28 July 1989):A5–A6.

Smeeding, Timothy, et al., eds. *Should Medical Care be Rationed by Age?* Totowa, New Jersey: Rowman & Littlefield, 1987.

Smith, Lawrence. "The Battle Over Health Insurance," *Fortune* (26 Sept. 1988):145–150.

Sobel, Lester, ed. *Health Care: An American Crisis*. New York: Facts on File, Inc., 1976.

Sonnefeld, Sally, Daniel Waldo, Jeffrey Lemieux, and David McKusick. "Projections of Health Care Spending Through the Year 2000," *Health Care Financing Review* 13(1):1–27 HCFA Pub. No. 03321. Washington, D.C.: HCFA, 1991.

"Sources Of Information In International Benefits." *Interben* 6 (July 1988):Supp. 4 pp.

"State Laws Regarding AIDS Include Restrictions for Testing, Insurance, Confidentiality." *Spencer's Research Reports on Employee Benefits* (Dec. 1987):325–327.

"State-Mandated Coverages Add To Costs, Make Policies Unaffordable By Uninsured." *Benefits Today* (16 Dec. 1988):409.

Steinwald, Bruce and Laura Dummit. "Hospital Case-Mix Change: Sicker Patients or DRG Creep?" *Health Affairs* (Summer 1989):35–47.

Sullivan, Cynthia and Thomas Rice. "The Health Insurance Picture in 1990," *Health Affairs* (Summer 1991):104–115.

Summers, Lawrence H. "What Can Economics Contribute to Social Policy?" *American Economic Review* (May 1989):177–183.

"Survey Search: Consumers and Employers on Long-Term Care." *Health Cost Management* 4 (July/Aug. 1987):28–33.

Swartz, Katherine. "Why Requiring Employers to Provide Health Insurance is a Bad Idea," *Journal of Health Politics, Policy and Law* (Winter 1990):779–792.

Swartz, Marvin. "Why Requiring Employers to Provide Health Insurance is a Bad Idea," *Journal of Health Politics, Policy and Law* 151(1990):779–792.

Sweeney, John. "National Health Care Reform—A Labor Perspective," *Employee Benefits Digest*, International Foundation of Employee Benefit Plans (February 1991):1, 8.

Tallon, James, Jr. "A Health Policy Agenda Proposal for Including the Poor," *Journal of the American Medical Association* 261 (1989):1044.

Taravella, Steve. "Coping With AIDS: Employers Tout Case Management," *Business Insurance* 21 (7 Sept. 1987):1, 20, 22.

"Tax-Favored Prefunding Of Retiree Plans Unlikely." *Employee Benefit Plan Review* (Aug. 1989):38–39.

Taylor, Malcolm. *Health Insurance and Canadian Public Policy: The Seven Decisions That Created the Canadian Health Insurance System*. Montreal: McGill-Queen's University Press, 1978.

Taylor, Malcolm. *Health Insurance and Canadian Public Policy: The Seven Decisions That Created the Canadian Health Insurance System and Their Outcomes* 2d ed. Toronto: Institute of Public Administration of Canada, 1987.

Thomas, J. W. and R. L. Lichtenstein. "Functional Health Measure For Adjusting Health Maintenance Organization Capitation Rates," *Health Care Financing Review* (Spring 1986):85–95.

Thompson, Roger. "Curbing The High Cost Of Health Care," *Nation's Business* (September 1989):1–8.

Thompson, Roger. "A NO to National Health Insurance," *Nation's Business* (May 1990):60.

Thorpe, Kenneth and Joanna Siegel. "Covering the Uninsured: Interactions Among Public and Private Sector Strategies," *Journal of the American Medical Association* 262 (October 1989):2114–2118.

U.S. Chamber of Commerce. *1990 Analysis of Workers Compensation Laws*. Washington, D.C.: U.S. Chamber of Commerce, 1991.

U.S. Department of Commerce. *Statistical Abstract of the United States 1991*. Washington, D.C.: Bureau of the Census, 1991.

U.S. Dept. of Health and Human Services. *The Medicare Handbook*. Baltimore: Health Care Financing Administration, 1989.

U.S. Dept. of Health and Human Services. *GUIDE: To Health Insurance for People with Medicare, 1990*. Baltimore: Health Care Financing Administration, 1990.

U.S. Dept. of Labor. *Employee Benefits in Medium and Large Firms, 1989*, Bulletin 2363. Washington, D.C.: Bureau of Labor Statistics, 1990.

U.S. Dept. of Labor. *Fiduciary Standards Employee Retirement Income Security Act*. Washington, D.C.: Labor-Management Services Administration, 1989.

U.S. Dept. of Labor. *What You Should Know About the Pension Law*. Washington, D.C.: Pension and Welfare Benefits Administration, 1988.

U.S. House of Representatives. *Medicare Long-Term Care Catastrophic Protection Act*, 100th Cong., 24 June 1987, H.R. 2762.

U.S. House of Representatives. *Long Term Home Care Act of 1988*, 101st Cong., 2nd Sess., 1988, H.R. 2263.

U.S. House of Representatives. *Long-Term Strategies For Health Care*, Hearings Before the Committee on Ways and Means, House of Representatives, Serial 102–33, 102d Cong., 1st Sess., April 16–17, 23–25, 1991. Washington, D.C.: U.S. Government Printing Office, 1991, pp. 374–403.

U.S. House of Representatives. *Oversight Hearing on National Health Care Reform*, Serial No. 102–104, 7 May 1992. Washington, D.C.: U.S. Government Printing Office, 1992.

U.S. House of Representatives, Energy and Commerce Subcommittee on Health and the Environment. *Elder-Care Long-Term Care Assistance Act of 1988*, 100th Cong., 16 September 1988, H.R. 5320.

U.S. House of Representatives, Select Committee on Aging. *Building An American Health*

System: Journey Toward A Healthy And Caring America, Comm. Pub. No. 101–740, 101st Cong., Jan. 1990.

U.S. House of Representatives, Ways and Means Subcommittee on Health. *Chronic Care Medicare Long-Term Care Coverage Act of 1988*, 100th Cong., 27 September 1988, H.R. 5393.

U.S. Senate, Finance Subcommittee on Health. *Long-Term Care Assistance Act*, 100th Cong., 21 April 1988, S. 2305.

U.S. Senate, Labor and Human Resources Subcommittee on Health. *Life-Care Long-Term Care Protection Act*, 100th Cong., 3 August 1988, S. 2681.

Vihtelic, J. "Allocating Child Care Expenses Between a Salary Reduction Plan and the Tax Credit," *Taxes* (Feb. 1989):83–87.

Wagner, Lynn. "National Health Plan Opposed," *Modern Healthcare* (2 April 1990):4.

Wallack, Stanley, Christopher Tompkins, and Leonard Gruenberg. "A Plan For Rewarding Efficient HMOs," *Health Affairs* (Summer 1988):80–96.

Walsh, Diana et al. "Posthospital Convalescence And Return To Work," *Health Affairs* (Fall 1989):76–90.

Weatherington, Richard. "A Promise Not Kept," *Modern Maturity* (June–July 1990):30–38.

Weber, David. "Data Bank, Heal Thyself," *Insurance Review* (September 1991):47–50.

Weber, Joseph et al. "The Price Of No-Name Drugs May Soon Be Hard To Swallow," *Business Week* (2 Oct. 1989):87.

Weiss, S. "Health Care Costs . . . A National Crisis," *NEA Today* (April 1990):10–11.

Weissert, William, Cynthia Cready, and James Pawelak. "The Past And Future Of Home- And Community-Based Long-Term Care," *The Milbank Quarterly* 66:2 (1988):309–388.

Welch, Pete. "Prospective Payment To Medical Staffs: A Proposal," *Health Affairs* (Spring 1989):34–49.

Weller, Geoffrey. "Common Problems, Alternative Solutions: A Comparison of the Canadian and American Health Systems," *Policy Studies Journal* (June 1986):604–620.

West, Jane. "Introduction—Implementing the Act: Where We Begin," *The Milbank Quarterly* Supp. 1/2, 69 (1991):xi–xxxi.

West, Jane, ed. *The Americans with Disabilities Act: From Policy to Practice*. New York, Milbank Memorial Fund, 1991.

West, Jane, ed. "The Social and Policy Context of the Act" in *The Americans with Disabilities Act: From Policy to Practice*. New York, Milbank Memorial Fund, 1991:3–24.

Westerfield, Donald L. "Degenerative Patterns in Health Disaggregation," *Health Care Administration Proceedings of the Midwest Business Administration Association* (Mar. 1987):89–91.

Westerfield, Donald L. "Public Welfare Strategies Related to Patients With AIDS/HIV," Fifteenth Annual Meeting of the Midsouth Academy of Economics and Finance, Hot Springs, (Feb. 17–20, 1988).

Westerfield, Donald L. "Analysis of Cost in Regulating and Treating AIDS and Related Diseases," *Proceedings of the 1988 Conference of the Business and Health Administration Association* (Mar. 1988):132–137.

Westerfield, Donald L. "Practices In Restraint Of Trade In The Health Care Industry," Twenty-Fourth Annual Meeting of the Missouri Valley Economic Association, Saint Louis, March 10–12, 1988.

Westerfield, Donald. *Mandated Health Care: Issues and Strategies*. New York: Praeger Publishers, 1991.

Westerfield, Donald L. and James Brasfield. "Analysis of Long Term Health Care Strategies," *Proceedings of the 1988 Conference of the Business and Health Administration Association* (Mar. 1988):150–156.

Westerfield, Donald L. and James Brasfield. "Assessing the Incidence of Long Term Health Care," Presented at The Southwestern Economic Association, March 29– April 1, 1989, Little Rock.

Westerfield, Donald L., Honorable T. Curtis, A. Curtis, and T. Allen. "Prospective Reimbursement Plan for Long-Term Care," Presented at The Southwestern Economic Association, March 29–April 1, 1989, Little Rock.

Westerfield, Donald L., Honorable T. Curtis, A. Curtis, and T. Allen. "Prospective Reimbursement Plan for Long-Term Care: A State Model," *Southwestern Journal of Economic Abstracts* 10 (Nov. 1989):37–38.

Westerfield, Donald L. and Paul Wilson. "Post-Retirement Health Care: An Economic and Political Time Bomb," *Proceedings of the 1988 Conference of the Business and Health Administration Association* (Mar. 1988):204–209.

Westerfield, Donald L. and Paul Wilson. "COBRA Strikes Business in the Jugular," *Management Accounting* (Jan. 1989):36–38.

Westerfield, Donald L. and Paul Wilson. "COBRA's Hidden Tax on Employers: Compliance Strategies," *Southwestern Journal of Economic Abstracts* 10 (Nov. 1989):83–84.

Westerfield, Donald L. and Paul Wilson. "FASB 81—Prefunded Retiree Benefits Nightmare," *Controllers Quarterly* 5 (Mar. 1990):25–28.

Westerfield, Donald and Paul Wilson. "Coping with Federal and State Government Health Care Mandates: Employer Strategies," *Proceedings of the Business and Health Administration Association* (April 1991):12–17.

Westerfield, Donald and Paul Wilson. "Employers and the Medicare Secondary Payer: IRS/SSA/HCFA Data Match Project," *Proceedings of the Business and Health Administration Association* (March 1992):127–130.

White-Means, Shelley and Thornton, Michael. "Nonemergency Visits To Hospital Emergency Rooms: A Comparison Of Blacks And Whites," *The Milbank Quarterly* 67:1 (1989):35–57.

Wiener, Joshua and Rose Rubin. "The Potential Impact Of Private Long-Term Care Financing Options On Medicaid: The Next Thirty Years," *Journal Of Health Politics, Policy And Law* 14:2 (Summer 1989):327–340.

Wilensky, Gail. "The Real Price Of Mandating Health Benefits," *Business And Health* (Mar. 1989):32, 34–37.

Wilensky, Gail. "Cost Containment Overview," *Health Care Financing Review: 1991 Annual Supplement*. Baltimore, Maryland: Health Care Financing Administration, 1991.

Wilson, Paul and Donald Westerfield. "Is Shifting Health Care Costs the Right Strategy for the U.S.?" *NAEDA Journal* (December 1990):9–12.

Wing, Kenneth. *The Law and the Public's Health* 3rd ed. Ann Arbor, Michigan: Health Administration Press, 1990.

Wolman, William, ed. "The Top 200: Who's Who Among Corporate Pension Funds," *Business Week* (6 Nov. 1989):174.

Woolsey, Christine. "Not Ready to Give Up: Employers Still Want to Provide Health Coverage," *Business Insurance* (20 May 1991):3.

Yelin, Edward. "The Recent History and Immediate Future of Employment among Persons with Disabilities" in Jane West, ed., *The Americans with Disabilities Act: From Policy to Practice*. New York, Milbank Memorial Fund, 1991:129–149.

Young, Casey and Phillip Polakoff. "Beyond Workers' Compensation: A New Vision," *Benefits Quarterly* (3rd Quarter 1992):56–65.

Zedlewski, Sheila. *Expanding the Employer-Provided Health Insurance System: Effects on Workers and Their Employers*, Urban Institute Report 91–3. Washington, D.C.: Urban Institute Press, 1991.

Zedlewski, Sheila, Gregory Acs, and Colin Winterbottom. "Play-or-Pay Employer Mandates: Potential Effects," *Health Affairs* (Spring 1992):62–83.

Zellers, Wendy, Catherine McLaughlin, and Kevin Frick. "Small-Business Health Insurance: Only Healthy Need Apply," *Health Affairs* (Spring 1992):174–180.

U.S. HOUSE OF REPRESENTATIVES BILLS

U.S. House of Representatives. "Civil Rights and Women's Equity in Employment Act of 1991," H.R. 1, 102d Cong., 1st Sess. (Washington, D.C.: U.S. Government Printing Office, 1991).

U.S. House of Representatives. "Comprehensive Health Care for All Americans Act" "(Claude Pepper Comprehensive Health Care Act)" H.R. 8, 102d Cong., 1st Sess. (Washington, D.C.: U.S. Government Printing Office, 1991).

U.S. House of Representatives. "National Health Insurance Act," H.R. 16, 102d Cong., 1st Sess. (Washington, D.C.: U.S. Government Printing Office, 1991).

U.S. House of Representatives. "MediPlan Act of 1991," H.R. 650, 102d Cong., 1st Sess. (Washington, D.C.: U.S. Government Printing Office, 1991).

U.S. House of Representatives. "Pepper Commission Health Care Access and Reform Act of 1991," H.R. 1177, 102d Cong., 1st Sess. (Washington, D.C.: U.S. Government Printing Office, 1991).

U.S. House of Representatives. "HealthAmerica: Affordable Health Care for All Americans Act," H.R. 1227, 102d Cong., 1st Sess. (Washington, D.C.: U.S. Government Printing Office, 1991).

U.S. House of Representatives. "Universal Health Care Act of 1991," H.R. 1300, 102d Cong., 1st Sess. (Washington, D.C.: U.S. Government Printing Office, 1991).

U.S. House of Representatives. "Universal Health Care Act of 1991," H.R. 1300, 102d Cong., 2nd Sess. (Washington, D.C.: U.S. Government Printing Office, 1992).

U.S. House of Representatives. "Medicare Universal Coverage Expansion Act of 1991," H.R. 1777, 102d Cong., 1st Sess. *Congressional Record—Extension of Remarks* (16 April 1991):E1261–E1262.

U.S. House of Representatives. "Better Access to Affordable Health Care Act of 1991,"
    H.R. 1872, 102d Cong., 1st Sess. (Washington, D.C.: U.S. Government Printing
    Office, 1991).
U.S. House of Representatives. "Health Equity and Access Improvement Act of 1991,"
    H.R. 1936, 102d Cong., 1st Sess. (Washington, D.C.: U.S. Government Printing
    Office, 1991).
U.S. House of Representatives. "Comprehensive Health Insurance Plan of 1991," H.R.
    2114, 102d Cong., 1st Sess. (Washington, D.C.: U.S. Government Printing Of-
    fice, 1991).
U.S. House of Representatives. "Health Insurance Reform Act of 1991," H.R. 2121,
    102d Cong., 1st Sess. (Washington, D.C.: U.S. Government Printing Office,
    1991).
U.S. House of Representatives. "State Health Reform Opportunity Act of 1991," H.R.
    2297, 102d Cong., 1st Sess. (Washington, D.C.: U.S. Government Printing Of-
    fice, 1991).
U.S. House of Representatives. "Small Employer Health Insurance Incentive Act Of
    1991," H.R. 2453, 102d Cong., 1st Sess. (Washington, D.C.: U.S. Government
    Printing Office, 1991).
U.S. House of Representatives. "National Health Care and Cost Containment Act,"
    H.R. 2530, 102d Cong., 1st Sess. (Washington, D.C.: U.S. Government Printing
    Office, 1991).
U.S. House of Representatives. "Pepper Commission Health Care Access and Reform
    Act of 1991," H.R. 2535, 102d Cong., 1st Sess. (Washington, D.C.: U.S.
    Government Printing Office, 1991).
U.S. House of Representatives. "Health Care Liability Reform and Quality of Care
    Improvement Act of 1991," H.R. 3037, 102d Cong., 1st Sess. (Washington,
    D.C.: U.S. Government Printing Office, 1991).
U.S. House of Representatives. "Health Insurance Coverage and Cost Containment Act
    of 1991," H.R. 3205, 102d Cong., 1st Sess. (Washington, D.C.: U.S. Govern-
    ment Printing Office, 1991).
U.S. House of Representatives. "USHealth Program Act of 1991," H.R. 3535, 102d
    Cong., 2nd Sess. (Washington, D.C.: U.S. Government Printing Office, 1992).
U.S. House of Representatives. "Health Insurance Reform and Cost Control Act of
    1991," H.R. 3626, 102d Cong., 2nd Sess. (Washington, D.C.: U.S. Government
    Printing Office, 1992).
U.S. House of Representatives. "To Repeal the Americans with Disabilities Act of 1990,"
    H.R. 5450, 102d Cong., 2nd Sess. (Washington, D.C.: U.S. Government Printing
    Office, 1992).
U.S. House of Representatives. "Health Care Cost Containment and Reform Act of
    1992," H.R. 5502, 102d Cong., 2nd Sess. (Washington, D.C.: U.S. Government
    Printing Office, 1992).

U.S. SENATE BILLS

U.S. Senate. "Comprehensive Health Care Act of 1991," S. 314, 102d Cong., 1st Sess.
    (Washington, D.C.: U.S. Government Printing Office, 1991).

U.S. Senate. "Health Care Act," S. 454, 102d Cong., 1st Sess. (Washington, D.C.: U.S. Government Printing Office, 1991).

U.S. Senate. "American Health Security Act of 1991," S. 700, 102d Cong., 1st Sess. (Washington, D.C.: U.S. Government Printing Office, 1991).

U.S. Senate. "Health Care Liability Reform and Quality Care Improvement Act of 1991," S. 1123, 102d Cong., 1st Sess. (Washington, D.C.: U.S. Government Printing Office, 1991).

U.S. Senate. "Pepper Commission Health Care Access and Reform Act of 1991," S. 1177, 102d Cong., 1st Sess. (Washington, D.C.: U.S. Government Printing Office, 1991).

U.S. Senate. "Medicaid Glideslope Act of 1991," S. 1211, 102d Cong., 1st Sess. (Washington, D.C.: U.S. Government Printing Office, 1991).

U.S. Senate. "HealthAmerica: Affordable Health Care for All Americans Act," S. 1227, 102d Cong., 1st Sess. (Washington, D.C.: U.S. Government Printing Office, 1991).

U.S. Senate. "Small Employer Health Insurance Incentive Act of 1991," S. 1229, 102d Cong., 1st Sess. (Washington, D.C.: U.S. Government Printing Office, 1991).

U.S. Senate. "Health USA Act of 1991," S. 1446, 102d Cong., 1st Sess. (Washington, D.C.: U.S. Government Printing Office, 1991).

U.S. Senate. "Improvements to the HealthAmerica Act of 1991," S. 1669, 102d Cong., 1st Sess. (Washington, D.C.: U.S. Government Printing Office, 1991).

U.S. Senate. "Better Access to Affordable Health Care Act of 1991," S. 1872, 102d Cong., 1st Sess. (Washington, D.C.: U.S. Government Printing Office, 1991).

U.S. Senate. "Health Equity and Access Improvement Act of 1991," S. 1936, 102d Cong., 1st Sess. (Washington, D.C.: U.S. Government Printing Office, 1991).

U.S. Senate. "State Care: State-Based Comprehensive Health Care Act of 1991," S. 1972, 102d Cong., 1st Sess. (Washington, D.C.: U.S. Government Printing Office, 1991).

U.S. Senate. "Health Care Access and Affordability Act of 1991," S. 1995, 102d Cong., 1st Sess. (Washington, D.C.: U.S. Government Printing Office, 1991).

U.S. Senate. "Access to Health Care for All Americans Act of 1991," S. 2036, 102d Cong., 1st Sess. (Washington, D.C.: U.S. Government Printing Office, 1991).

U.S. Senate. "Comprehensive Health Insurance Plan of 1991 (CHIP of 1991)," S. 2114, 102d Cong., 1st Sess. (Washington, D.C.: U.S. Government Printing Office, 1991).

Index

ABOUT THE AUTHOR

DONALD L. WESTERFIELD is a Professor in the Graduate School of Webster University in St. Louis, Missouri. He is the author of *Mandated Health Care* (Praeger, 1991) and co-author (with Thomas Curtis) of *Congressional Intent* (Praeger, 1992).